Vocational and Personal Adjustments in Practical Nursing

Vocational and Personal Adjustments in Practical Nursing

BETTY GLORE BECKER, RN, BS

Evening Supervisor, Our Lady of Victories;
formerly Staff Nurse, Our Lady of Victories;
formerly Assistant Director of Nurses, St. Louis County Hospital;
Instructor, Community School of Practical Nursing,
St. Louis-Little Rock Hospital;
Day Surgical Supervisor, St. Louis-Little Rock Hospital;
Head Nurse, Missouri Pacific Hospital;
Assistant Head Nurse, Missouri Pacific Hospital;
Staff Nurse, Missouri Pacific Hospital, St. Louis, Missouri

DOLORES T. FENDLER, RN, BSN, MEd

Formerly Director of School of Practical Nursing, St. Mary's Health Center;
Assistant Director and Surgical Instructor,
School of Practical Nursing, St. Mary's Health Center;
Group Nurse, St. Mary's Health Center and Deaconess Hospital;
Staff Nurse, Surgical Intensive Care Unit,
St. Mary's Health Center, St. Louis, Missouri;
Staff Nurse, Obstetrical Unit, Mercy Hospital,
San Diego, California

SEVENTH EDITION

with illustrations

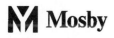 Mosby

An Affiliate of Elsevier Science

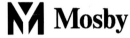 **Mosby**

An Affiliate of Elsevier Science

SEVENTH EDITION
Copyright © 1994 by Mosby , Inc.

Previous editions copyrighted

Printed in the United States of America

Mosby , Inc.
11830 Westline Industrial Drive
St. Louis, Missouri 63146

Library of Congress Cataloging in Publication Data

Becker, Betty Glore.
    Vocational and personal adjustments in practical nursing / Betty
Glore Becker, Dolores T. Fendler.—7th ed.
        p.   cm.
    Includes bibliographical references and index.
    ISBN 0-8016-6839-5
    1. Practical nursing. 2. Student adjustment. 3. Practical
nursing—Vocational guidance. I. Fendler, Dolores T.
II. Title.
    [DNLM: 1. Nursing, Practical. WY 195 B395v 1993]
RT62.B43 1993
610.73'06'93—dc20
DNLM/DLC   93-8185

02 03 / 9 8 7 6 5

Contributors

MARY ROOT, RN, BSN, MS, MSN

Faculty
Associate Degree Nursing Program
Madison Area Technical College
Madison, Wisconsin

MARY ANN SHEA, RN, ATTORNEY AT LAW

Medical/Legal Consultant
St. Louis, Missouri

GLORIA E. WOLD, RN, BSN, MS

Instructor/Lab Manager
Milwaukee Area Technical College
Milwaukee, Wisconsin

Reviewers

DAWN E. BLEAU, RN

Director
Knoedler School of Practical Nursing Education
Jefferson, Ohio

PATTI POND SCOTT, RN

Kilgore College
Longview, Texas

JUDY WENLAND, RN, MED, MSN

LVN Program Director
Mount San Jacinto Community College
San Jacinto, California

To the Instructor

This book has been compiled to assist you in helping students make the necessary professional and personal adjustments inherent in their development as practical nurses. The informal style is designed to capture student interest and enliven factual material to facilitate understanding and retention. We have attempted to pinpoint student ideas and feelings in stated situations; to offer positive suggestions for initiating changes when necessary; to provide basic principles needed for physical, psychological, social, and religious interactions and behavior; to outline systematic plans to implement these principles; and to provide organizational structures and functions that affect and involve practical nurses.

Our expectation in providing you with this book is that it will be a helpful resource in accomplishing your instructional goals. However, it is valueless if you do not have a clear understanding of nursing, of current knowledge of the functions and changes initiated by advances in technology, of societal needs and projects, of the importance and role of the practical nurse as a member of the health team, and of the opportunities available for advancement of practical nurses. Students will look to you for more complete knowledge and practical application of principles described in this book. Unless you can demonstrate that you are a "living image" of these principles, students will be slow to grasp and incorporate them into their personal and professional lifestyles. No book can be a substitute for the *real* you as seen in the ever-watchful eyes of your students.

The terms *practical* and *vocational* nurse are used synonymously in this book. Because the majority of states use the term *practical,* we have generally followed this practice. The practical nurse is referred to as "she," but we recognize the male nurses in the profession. We have attempted to show the relationship between familiar animate and inanimate objects with less tangible traits and characteristics. These relationships should further students' learning abilities and powers to transfer knowledge into meaningful expressions. If knowledge has true meaning for students, they will grasp, retain, and use it in their developmental process.

As with previous editions, we have made an effort to identify and clarify those issues and trends in the health care system that affect practical nursing.

New to this edition are sections on the care of AIDS patients, some advantages and disadvantages of practicing in home health and the hospice unit, and revisions throughout the chapters, including a new chapter on legal aspects and the practical nurse. We believe these issues to be of vital concern to all health care professionals but of particular relevance to the practice and future of practical nursing.

Visually realistic photographs and artwork have been selected to illustrate situations as they are today in the health care world.

It is our hope that this book will assist you in making your course interesting, alive, and valuable to your students.

We express our sincere appreciation for the interest, encouragement, and assistance we have received from Dolores' husband, Kermit F. Fendler, graduates of St. Mary's Health Center and the former Community School of Practical Nursing, and family, and friends.

Betty Glore Becker
Dolores T. Fendler

To the Student

The purpose of this book is to help you to understand yourself, to develop your traits to their fullest potential, and to alter and rechannel your less desirable characteristics. The book provides you with positive suggestions for needed change, supplies guidelines for personal and professional behavior and activities, and establishes the necessary requisites inherent in your profession as a practical nurse. It discloses opportunities, organizational structures, and commitments in which you are or will be involved.

In writing this seventh edition, we have tried to incorporate the constructive suggestions and comments of many readers and reviewers so that the book will be more helpful.

Because the profession you have chosen demands knowledgeable practitioners, individual responsibility and specific modes of action are necessary. Through knowledge, awareness, and responsibility, you will be able to develop maturity, which is essential in a practical nurse.

This book is written in an informal style with the hope that you will find the material interesting, informative, and meaningful, thus making it a part of yourself. The practical nurse is referred to as "she," but we recognize the male nurses in the profession. Your future must be founded on a firm, broad foundation if you are to build on it throughout life. The challenge is yours! Your instructors, with the aid of textbooks, can point the way, but they cannot force you to follow given directions. You must choose for yourself. This book will assist you in overcoming obstacles and in making adjustments; it will supply you with knowledge, methods, and principles basic to your profession. By studying the materials and applications, your task will be easier and your adjustment smoother. Remember, this book is only a tool, not an end. If you use if carefully, conscientiously, and with determination, you will succeed in transforming yourself from an untrained student into a skilled licensed practical nurse.

Betty Glore Becker
Dolores T. Fendler

Contents

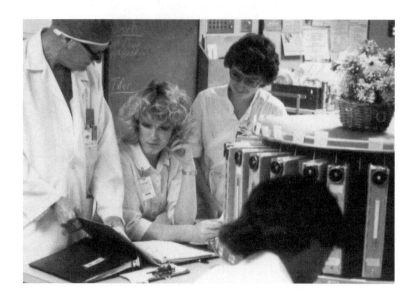

Objectives

At the completion of this chapter the student practical nurse will be able to:

♦ Discuss ways to study smarter, not harder.

♦ Describe the process of communication.

♦ Explain the five steps in problem solving.

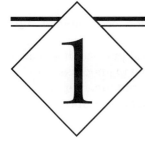

Practical Nursing as an Educational Program

◆ Educational Program

Some of the days you will long remember are those spent as a practical nurse. You have chosen a career that presents many challenges and requires much discipline, a career to serve the best interests of self and society. The following months will be filled with much work and study; however, when you complete the course, you will experience a sense of fulfillment and pride in your achievement.

An orientation period may be scheduled before the formal beginning of classes or on the first day of class. At this time faculty members meet with students to review the philosophy and objectives of the program, review the rules and regulations of the program, and acquaint the students with the physical facilities in which they will function.

Faculties in schools of practical nursing have a strong commitment to you, the student, and make every effort to assure your success in the program. The practical nursing program is planned to incorporate basic principles with practical experience in a 1-year period. Principles underlying each procedure precede its practice. It is important for the patient's welfare and for the development of the learning process to know not only *how* to perform a procedure but also *why* you are doing it. The *why* is presented to you in lecture sessions, and the *how*, in laboratory demonstrations.

Practical nursing programs are designed in various ways to incorporate lecture with practice. Following are some practical nursing programs:

1. Courses in basic principles given in a 16- to 20-week preclinical period with applied practice in the remaining clinical period (32 to 36 weeks); advanced courses given concurrently with specific clinical areas.
2. Courses in basic and advanced concepts given concurrently with practical application during each rotation in clinical areas.
3. Lectures given at a junior college with clinical practice in affiliated institutions (for example, hospitals, nursing homes, and community health programs).

Basic courses may be given during a preclinical period or combined with advanced principles during specific clinical rotations.

4. Theory given in a vocational technical school with clinical practice in affiliated institutions. The program of instruction is the same as that in junior colleges.

Basic curriculum includes communications, body structure and function, pharmacology, solutions and dosages, professional adjustments, fundamentals of nursing, mental health, geriatrics, and nutrition and diet therapy. These studies can be applied to all clinical areas. Advanced instruction includes scientific principles, nursing skills, and procedures specific to clinical areas such as obstetrics, psychiatry, orthopedics, medical-surgical nursing, and pediatrics.

◆ Adjustments to Student Life

In addition to the instructional program, student life requires making adjustments to school rules and regulations; to a hospital–medical center environment; to the personalities of various members of the medical team, patients, and family members; and to all the drama, trauma, joy, and sorrow found in a hospital.

Student Counseling

In most schools of practical nursing, faculty members counsel students to ensure academic and professional success. Counseling sessions may be scheduled on a biweekly or bimonthly basis, on an individual basis at the discretion of the faculty member, or from a personal request of the student. Faculty members may direct the student to a professional counselor, often assisting with arrangements, giving encouragement, and communicating with the counselor so the student may obtain the needed guidance.

Study Habits

The following suggestions may help you to study smarter, not harder.

Study ahead of time. Avoid waiting until the day before the test to study. Through study, you understand the information and are better prepared to take the test. Use the day before the test to review.

Avoid distractions. Close doors to diminish noise. Before you begin to study, tend to your physical needs.

Gather materials. Have available sharp pencils, a dictionary, books, notebook, eraser, and colored marker for highlighting important phrases, ideas, and principles you want to remember.

Reward yourself. Reward yourself only after you have completed the task.

Be confident. Believe that you can and will learn the material.

Scan. Scan the unit or chapter you are about to read. Ask yourself the following questions:

1. What is the chapter about?
2. What are the main sections of the chapter?
3. Is there a word glossary?
4. Are there questions at the end of the chapter?
5. What do the graphs and illustrations indicate?

Measure. After scanning the chapter, make an assessment of the amount of work and material involved. Be realistic. If there is more material than you can finish in one study session, set a definite time for a second study session.

Look ahead. Read each heading. Understand information given and make up questions you will answer later.

Read and review. Read one section at a time, and answer the questions you formulated. Review all the information in one section, and be certain you understand the information before proceeding to the next section.

Trace. Examine what you have read. Do you remember the major heading? Are you able to answer the questions at the end of the chapter or unit? Can you define words in the glossary? Are there portions of the chapter you need to review? If so, review and understand before you go on. This technique is also useful as a study review the night before a test.

Take notes. Use *color coding,* yellow or green for highlighting and red for important items. Use *flip words.* These are words written on corners or insides of pages that call your attention to important phrases or statements. Use *abbreviations;* however, be sure you understand what the abbreviations mean. Use *main headings.* Write notes beneath headings in outline form. Do not write down information you already know. Use complete sentences wherever necessary. *Review* your notes as soon as possible. Remember, much of what is forgotten is forgotten within 24 hours after having been read or heard.

◆ Communication Skills

Communication is not simply sending a message; it is creating true understanding swiftly, clearly, and precisely. In communication, ideas need to travel between the sender and the receiver. The sender is the speaker or writer; the receiver is the listener or the reader. If communication is to be productive, the receiver must comprehend the message the sender is trying to convey.

We must communicate to survive. People depend on other people to meet many of their physiologic needs, such as food, water, shelter, and clothing; their environmental needs, such as electricity, cars, and telephones; and their emotional needs, such as feeling secure, belonging, and being somebody. Think of what it would be like if we had no automobiles, no clean water, no electricity, and no hospitals. The idea is difficult to conceive because we have become accustomed to these comforts. We forget that these comforts originated with someone's ideas and that many people worked together to make them realities.

The ability or inability to communicate affects our relationships with people. Language and communication are interrelated. Try thinking about what you will wear to a party this weekend. Your thoughts entailed words, didn't they?

If someone speaks to you, the sounds become words and you mentally entertain certain ideas. The sender changes these ideas into words and the receiver changes these words back into ideas. If the sender's message matches the idea of the receiver, communication takes place. If not, a breakdown in communication occurs.

Through language, humans are able to express themselves and satisfy their needs and desires. Through communication, people are able to live, work, and play together. The art of communication involves the use of taste, touch, smell, sight, and hearing; in many cases several of these are used simultaneously. For instance, imagine being complimented verbally on your appearance by a person whose eyes tell you he does not mean what he is saying. In such a case you have received two conflicting messages, one verbal and the other nonverbal. You exercise intelligence and experience to find out exactly what was being communicated. Have you ever found yourself sitting on the edge of your chair after telling someone that you were not in a hurry? This unconscious gesture communicates your real feelings more clearly than words. Have you ever caught yourself handling patients not quite as gently as you should because you disliked them, your supervisor, or yourself? Something about the touch of a human hand is soothing to people who are ill. The pressure applied should be smooth and gentle. If you are overly brisk, believing it to be a sign of efficiency, you impress no one; and your brisk, hasty, and agitated manner communicates to your patient and others your impatience and lack of caring. Watch carefully that your verbal and nonverbal messages do not contradict each other, because when they do, the nonverbal are the messages people believe.

Various factors may cause ineffective communication between you and your patient. If you state personal opinions, jump to conclusions, give inappropriate reassurance, change the subject, belittle the patient's feelings, or disapprove or disagree with him, communication is impaired. To develop effective techniques, you must be able to evaluate the individual situation and recognize the need to be observant and objective. Experience, time, and the assistance of your instructors will help you develop these techniques.

In nursing practice the importance of observation is constantly stressed because it enables nurses to be more sensitive "receivers" of nonverbal communication from their patients. In our society it has become an established norm to suppress as much as possible any show of emotion; therefore you find that patients may hesitate to tell you verbally about their fears, worries, or physical discomforts. But as an alert nurse you find they communicate to you by nonverbal messages. For example, patients may communicate physical discomfort by facial expressions and eye movements, agitation by restlessness, or fear by crying.

Being a good listener is required of every nurse. Listening is one part of observation. It is also important in developing complete confidence between nurse and patient, an essential therapeutic measure.

Hearing and listening are different. Hearing is being in the range of and receiving sound waves, whereas listening is the interpretation of spoken words. A person spends 70% of a day in communication. A person can speak 125 words per minute but think

400 to 700 words per minute. Seventy-five percent of oral communication is lost through poor listening. Listening demands a conscious effort on your part.

Listening well enables the patient to release emotional tension because talking is an active process. Encouraging patients to talk does not entitle you to probe into their personal lives. Be patient and receptive, but remember your role. Once patients suspect you of "invading" their thoughts, they probably will discontinue all communication with you.

Remember that listening to a patient is not the same as social conversation. When the patient tells of some significant experience, you should not relate a similar one of your own. Listen quietly, and if you need to express agreement, smile, nod your head, and respond to the cues, but do not interrupt. You may indicate to the patient that you have listened by asking questions or paraphrasing, but never probe.

If you listen carefully, you discover what people need, what they want, how they feel, and often what they are. Because every patient's situation is different, little advice can be included on *what* to say. The following suggestions for *how* you speak to a patient may be helpful.

If the hands are used to communicate, keep the palms open and upward. This expresses honesty. Acquire an appropriate vocabulary. This helps to avoid the use of wrong words, the omission of important ideas, and the use of long, rambling descriptions that often confuse rather than enlighten a patient. Learn to offer precise, accurate descriptions. Use words sparingly but wisely when communicating with patients or other health professionals. Use your own words to explain technical points to your patients in a simple manner. Speak clearly. An important sentence loses its meaning when poorly articulated or spoken too quickly or too softly. Many patients are too embarrassed to ask the nurse to repeat an instruction, so they try to decipher what they think they have heard. This causes a patient needless anxiety and results in unconventional behavior.

The quality of your voice is determined by your vocal cords, but your personality gives your voice an individuality that sets it apart from everyone else's. Words convey only one half of the message. Other variants—such as rhythm, stress, timing, tone, pause, pitch, and inflection—communicate subtler meanings. Because your voice tells much about you, concentrate on achieving control over it. Practice the art of communication with your classmates.

Organize your thoughts before addressing or answering a patient's questions. A health professional confuses a patient by jumping from one topic to another, interjecting last-minute ideas, and neglecting to either summarize or ask the patient to put into his own words what the nurse has said. Present a caring attitude. The attitude or feeling you express in your spoken interaction with your patient helps communicate genuine concern. Avoid saying the same thing to all patients because they sense that it is a memorized speech.

Verbal communication with members of the health team should be professional and exclude gossip and confidential information learned while caring for the patient, unless the coworker has a right to this information.

Written communication is frequently more important than verbal communication because of its far-reaching effects. It is often more accurate and thorough because it requires considerable thought, time, and energy. It also has greater legal implications.

Any written communication on a patient's chart is used not only to inform other members of the health team concerning the patient's progress but also as legal evidence in a court of law. Because the chart is a legal document, it may be used for or against you and the patient. This aspect alone warrants careful, thoughtful charting. Written communication is an effective means of communication, but it is dangerous if not learned and performed properly.

◆ Problem Solving

Life is full of problem situations, and the nursing profession is no exception. In your daily activities as a student practical nurse, you are faced with many problems. A *problem* can be defined as a lack of balance between the actual and the desired outcome that is of importance to people at a specific time and necessitates an improvement or solution.

You can become frustrated with problems or you can solve them, thus diminishing stress on yourself and others. Problem solving becomes an easier process if you choose a systematic approach.

The following approach may be helpful:

1. *Determine whether you have a problem.* To do this, ask yourself these questions:

   Why do I think I have a problem?

   What would happen if I did nothing about the problem?

   Why am I displeased or dissatisfied?

   If you determine that you have a problem, consider whether it is important enough to warrant further consideration. If not, ignore it. If so, proceed with the next series of steps.

2. *Determine the cause of the problem.*

   Gather together all pertinent data.

   Obtain facts from others and list the information gathered.

   Be objective and do not show partiality to any one person or group of facts.

   Examine the data and determine the cause of the problem.

   You may discover that the cause is a lack of knowledge, communication, or a specific skill; poor working relationships; personality conflicts, or that the issue has little meaning to the involved person.

3. *Outline possible solutions to the problem.* By listing specific causes, you determine possible solutions for each cause. The following are examples:

   If the cause is lack of knowledge, consider systematic practice or education.

   If the cause is punishing or nonrewarding consequences to the individual, provide favorable consequences and reduce or eliminate the negative effects.

   If the problem is the result of obstacles that prohibit performance, remove the obstacles.

   People perform or act in a certain manner because it has value for them.

   Determine the value that a particular action has for this person before trying to develop a workable solution.

4. *Choose and implement the best solution or solutions.*

Study the possible solutions that you have determined.

Do not rush to a solution before you have considered all elements of the problem.

In most situations you are dealing with infinitely variable entities—human beings—and although probably no perfect solution exists, some solutions are superior to others, and these are the solutions that should be chosen.

Concentrate on solutions directly related to the problem and choose from these.

Compare the size of the remedy (solution) to the size of the problem.

5. *Evaluate results.* After implementing the selected solution, be prepared to accept the consequences, good or bad. Evaluate results in terms of the following:

Was the solution effective? Did it solve the problem satisfactorily?

What were the shortcomings?

Could the problem have been solved more satisfactorily through the use of a different solution?

Although problem solving appears to be a long, drawn-out procedure, it can be accomplished in a relatively short time. The process is sensible and not too difficult. It requires you to thoroughly and clearly analyze difficult situations, called *problems.*

Student life is filled with adjustments, problems, interaction, responsibility, communication, study, and involvement. Each of these avenues causes you to grow in your personal and professional development. A systematic approach to problem solving aids you in knowing yourself better and in understanding your reactions to fears and problem situations. If you apply yourself earnestly in the beginning of the program, adjustments and solutions are made more easily and satisfactorily as you progress in your professional and personal career.

◆ *Study Helps*

1. Explain several methods used by practical nursing programs to incorporate theory with clinical practice.
2. List five good study habits.
3. Explain the process of communication.
4. What percent of communication is lost through poor listening?
5. List the three types of communication skills and briefly explain the purpose of each.
6. List and explain the five steps in problem solving.

Bibliography

Christensen B, Kockrow E: *Foundations of nursing,* ed 1, St Louis, 1991, Mosby.
Hill SS, Howlett HA: *Success in practical nursing,* ed 1, Philadelphia, 1988, WB Saunders.
Barkauskas V, Stoltenberg-Allen K: *Health assessment,* ed 5, St Louis, 1994, Mosby.

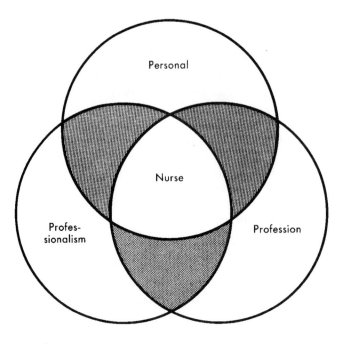

Objectives

At the completion of this chapter the student practical nurse will be able to:

◆ Define the term *profession.*

◆ Describe five types of posture.

◆ List five commonly abused drugs, their signs, and their effects.

◆ Define self-awareness.

◆ List ways in which the nurse assists the patient to adjust to a strange environment.

The Three Ps:

Profession, Person, Professionalism

◆ **Profession**

When someone speaks of a "new way of life," what immediately comes to your mind? Do you think of something different or challenging or of starting over?

You may regard practical nursing as a "new way of life." Practical nursing is an integral part of nursing and is the entry level into nursing. The educational program is taught in a vocational/technical school, junior college, or hospital. The vocational/technical program and the junior college program are usually government-funded. Hospital schools are generally departments of private hospitals, and maintenance of the school is included in the general budget of the hospital.

Practical nursing is an exciting and challenging career. It provides the opportunity to take care of others and receive personal gratification. Practical nurses function at the bedside of the patient, administering personal care in a variety of settings. To perform in a responsible and accountable manner the practical nurse must be skilled and knowledgeable.

The registered nurse is the direct health care giver. She practices in various settings and performs skills that are within the parameters and scope of the Nurse Practice Act of the state in which she practices.

A profession is defined as an occupation to which one devotes oneself and in which one has specialized expertise. The nurse is devoted to caring. She is strongly service-oriented and renders scientific and personal services to community members with specific health needs. Sacrifice, willingness, and selflessness are required. Through education and training, the nurse possesses specialized expertise. This expertise varies because the depth of theory taught at each level of nursing differs. The nurse has a profound concern for the welfare of others, in particular, those who suffer from illness or pain.

As you enter nursing, your "new way of life," the people who are closest to you are your fellow student nurses and your instructors. You come in contact with them before you reach the patient. You learn from them, with them, and through them. It is your opportunity to grow to your fullest and become a mature individual. Striving to know your companions, instructors, and yourself enables you to better understand the needs of your patients and to more easily administer quality patient care.

◆ Person

Self-Awareness

From childhood you have learned the basic needs of all humans: affection, success, and security. The manner in which each of these needs is met depends on the individual. People need to be loved and accepted by others. You may require more love than others, depending on your individual personality; however, you must give love before you can receive it. As a social being directly or indirectly responsible for the happiness of others, you are compelled to give this love to others. A person who loves is a generous, selfless person and thinks about another's welfare before his or her own. This person, although not expecting or demanding a return of love, cannot help but receive love or respect in return for generosity. The one who loves is a cherished friend on whom others depend to give a helping hand.

As a student you need the respect of your fellow students, instructors, patients, members of the medical team (although it may take time to establish this) and other hospital personnel. You want to be accepted and to feel as though you are part of each of these groups. Only in true acceptance can you find happiness in your profession. You can encourage this acceptance by learning and developing the qualifications, techniques, and skills that are essential in your professional and personal life.

Almost everyone wants success and achievement. There are degrees of achievement involving effort, perseverance, and challenge. The degree of accomplishment depends on the individual. Success in nursing depends on your efforts to study and learn about the profession and to apply these facts in practical situations. Because this process is full of trials and challenges, you must persevere in your efforts. If nursing had not presented a challenge to you, you would have sought another profession. A challenge spurs you to attempt to attain something that is out of your reach at the present time. The challenge is strengthened by your determination and your ideas. If you want to become a good nurse, you must not allow anything to interfere with your desire and goal.

If you are a stable individual, you feel secure. You are not swayed in any direction. However, this does not mean being stubborn or opinionated. You must know what to do, know how to do it, and have practice and experience in doing it. The more you do something, the more secure you feel in doing it. You must be willing to accept a better way of doing something if a better way becomes apparent, even though you may feel less secure at the beginning.

You cannot help others with problems if you do not recognize that you have problems. You must know what the problems and their possible solutions are and then choose and carry out the solutions. You need to understand your own reactions to various conditions and people. Only by controlling your feelings are you able to help others. For example, a patient becomes angry because he feels that he is receiving poor or insufficient nursing care. If you are the first person he encounters, he may begin to tell you in no uncertain terms his opinion about the hospital, the physician, the nursing staff, and perhaps you as an individual. Your reaction, if you are quick-tempered, may be to defend all involved, answering the patient in the same tone of voice he is using. However, if you know you have a quick temper, you can take positive steps to control it. In this instance you could count to 10 before you speak and could answer the patient kindly in a soft voice. You may tell the patient you are sorry that he feels this way and may try to determine what has happened to initiate the response. You may discover that the patient has been told by the physician that he has an incurable disease. The patient may not wish to accept this condition and may attempt to fight it by finding fault with the hospital, nursing personnel, and so on. If you become angry, you may never discover the patient's real problem and may fail to help him. You need to know yourself thoroughly to handle the patient's feelings.

Self-Esteem

Everyone has feelings about people, places, and things. These feelings may be positive or negative. They are positive if you seek the good in things, if you see life as worth living, and if you see it as something good and challenging. Love people and think kindly of them. Your friends and peers have faults, as you do, but their good qualities far exceed their less desirable characteristics. You have to believe that some things happen for good. Evil exists because there is a lack of goodness, but it gives you the opportunity to profit from another's mistakes as well as your own. Negative attitudes stifle your growth. They prevent you from accomplishing things you want to achieve. They make you sullen and lonely, because the negative person has few friends.

Mental health is something positive—peace of mind, happiness, enjoyment, and satisfaction from a job well done. It comes with satisfactory adjustment of your desires, ambitions, ideals, and feelings to the daily demands of living. Ordinarily mentally healthy people feel comfortable with themselves and others and are able to cope effectively with the demands of society. This includes the development of an open but analytic mind and shunning gossip and backbiting. Strive to see the good in others; stress good qualities rather than those less desirable. Help to develop friendships, and uphold your friends and their reputations. You are appreciated for your integrity and character as you do these things.

Appearance

Nurses are professional men and women. Their appearance, in addition to their actions and behavior, should attest to this. The appearance of the practical nurse should communicate a message of pride in oneself. To do this she must be clean and neatly dressed and have good posture. A clean nurse is free of body odor. Her hair is washed, combed, and neatly styled. Hair is best worn up and off the collar of the uniform and back from the face, so that when she is bending over the patient, it does not fall forward over her face. Hands and fingernails are especially important. Skin should be smooth and nails short to avoid scratching the patient. Excessive makeup and excessive jewelry are inappropriate to the nurse in uniform. Patients feel more comfortable with a neatly groomed nurse.

Posture

Posture indicates how we feel about ourselves. Different postures are associated with varying emotional tendencies. We usually think the person with an erect posture and squared shoulders is self-confident and capable. The person walking with shoulders bowed, head thrust forward, and eyes looking down communicates a lack of self-confidence and symbolizes a person carrying a heavy burden. An individual standing erect with hands on hips appears autocratic and dominant. Someone sitting with arms folded and shoulders curled inward portrays resignation and abandonment. A relaxed posture is a good indicator of feeling and status. Relaxed postures are evident in individuals having a conversation in which they share similar views. When you are with another person, your posture reflects your attitude toward that person. For this reason nurses must be particularly careful of the way they stand at the bedside of a patient. If their attitude is one of caring, their posture should be erect, not rigid; relaxed, not slouched; and positive, not submissive.

Health

Nutrition. The nurse must eat a regular and balanced diet to function properly and to keep physically fit. The nursing student is frequently a diet offender. She skips meals, eats improperly balanced diets, and follows crash diets. The student who skips breakfast for 10 minutes of extra sleep cannot function well. By midmorning she is frequently weak from hunger and unable to think correctly, thereby decreasing efficiency. This is a harmful practice. A good breakfast is a must if you are to perform nursing duties correctly and intelligently. Proper foods provide the nutrients and energy to carry out these activities.

The five basic food groups provide the foundation for selection of all nutrients required by the normal adult. The Recommended Dietary Allowances (RDAs) have been determined by a group of scientists to provide a margin of safety in the specified allowances to ensure maximum nutritional intake. Fats, oils, and sweets should be used sparingly in the diet. Excessive use of these increases the risk for obesity and coronary artery disease.

The following allowances are recommended for a normal American adult: 2 to 3 servings daily from the milk, yogurt, and cheese group; 2 to 3 servings from the meat, poultry, fish, dry beans, eggs, and nuts group; 3 to 5 servings from the vegetable group (for example, cabbage, carrots, and broccoli); 2 to 4 servings from the fruit group (for example, bananas, grapes, and oranges); and 6 to 11 servings from the bread, cereal, rice, and pasta group (see Fig. 2–1). Developing intelligent food habits founded on these basic food groups is one of the keys to your success as a student and as a licensed practical nurse.

We live in an impatient society. Most of us want instant results in anything we set out to do. When we decide to exercise, we want instantly to be fit. This leads to overexertion, pulled muscles, and aching joints and often forces us to give up our exercise program, at least temporarily.

When it comes to dieting, we decide how many pounds we want to lose and hope to lose them in a short period of time. Rapid weight loss leads to many of the following problems:

1. Organ mass decreases (especially in the lungs, heart, pancreas, spleen, liver, brain, and kidneys) and muscle mass decreases.
2. Almost all if not more of the weight that has been lost is often regained.
3. Infections occur often during and after rapid weight loss. This may be due to a decrease in the body's resistance to infections.

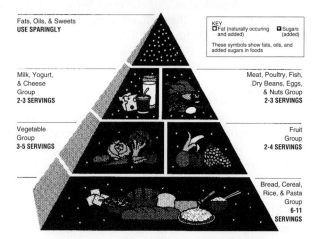

Food Guide Pyramid
A Guide to Daily Food Choices

Fats, Oils, & Sweets
USE SPARINGLY

KEY
☐ Fat (naturally occuring and added)   ☐ Sugars (added)
These symbols show fats, oils, and added sugars in foods

Milk, Yogurt, & Cheese Group
2-3 SERVINGS

Meat, Poultry, Fish, Dry Beans, Eggs, & Nuts Group
2-3 SERVINGS

Vegetable Group
3-5 SERVINGS

Fruit Group
2-4 SERVINGS

Bread, Cereal, Rice, & Pasta Group
6-11 SERVINGS

Fig. 2-1   U.S. Department of Agriculture, Washington, DC,1992.

4. Psychologic problems are common, ranging from depression to mania.
5. Bowel dysfunction, including persistent diarrhea, may result from losing weight too rapidly.

Except for people who are morbidly obese (100 lb or more overweight), a safe and better way to lose weight is at a rate of 2 lb per month, or 20 to 24 lb per year. To prevent weight from coming back you should weigh yourself everyday and average your weight every week. By looking from week to week you learn a great deal about yourself. If you gain 1 or 2 lb in a week, you can usually look back and figure out what caused it and eliminate it. Remember, to lose weight your calorie intake must be less than the amount lost in normal energy use. Weight reduction may occur as the result of eating balanced, nutritional meals in place of high-calorie meals and smaller amounts of food. Remember too, consult a physician before starting a strict reduction diet or exercise program.

Rest and sleep. Everyone needs sufficient rest and sleep to do a job well. The amount of sleep may vary with the individual. An infant or child requires more sleep than the young or middle-aged adult, who may need only 6 to 8 hours of sleep. Individual need is the determining factor of the amount of sleep required. Do not compare yourself with others. You may have a friend who requires only 5 hours of sleep. With this amount of sleep, this person functions without stress or strain. If you were to limit yourself to 5 hours of sleep when you need 8, this need would quickly manifest itself in your daily activities. You might show signs of fatigue, irritability, and lack of ambition. Your resistance to infection would be lessened. As a result you might suffer from frequent colds, the flu, or serious infections.

Sleep is a natural process and is essential to restore body powers. During the hours of sleep body parts are at their lowest ebb of functioning. They appear to be at a complete stage of rest or inactivity; however, complete inactivity cannot take place because body functions must continue to maintain life.

Rest is as important as sleep. Rest means the conscious freedom from activity. This rest can be mental, physical, or both. Physical rest means minimal activity of the body. Mental rest means minimal activity of the mind. If you are relaxed and are at peace with yourself, you are in a state of mental rest. There is no turmoil churning about in your mind. Rest requires the combination of physical and mental processes.

Tension. Tension is stress or the accumulation of inner pressures. It is caused by the conflict of two opposing forces. For example, a woman who is married to an alcoholic husband may try repeatedly to satisfy her husband in every way so that his need for alcohol is diminished. After repeated efforts without success, she may decide to leave him. What are the two opposing forces in this situation? One is the fact that she loves him and wants to help him. She married him for better or for worse and wants to fulfill her side of the marriage contract. The other is the fact that he refuses her help, and he mistreats her with verbal and physical attacks. Because she believes that she cannot withstand this treatment any longer, she leaves him. These two forces are raging within her, and only one can win. Either she remains with her alcoholic husband and suffers the abuse, or she leaves him. This conflict builds up emotional pressures within her. These pressures may appear in various physical symptoms such as headaches or pain. They may lead to the creation of a dream world and loss of contact with reality. She may find suitable outlets for these pressures through physical activities such as community organizations and activities, an exercise program, or just being able to speak privately to a person (a friend) she trusts.

As a student nurse, how do you cope with daily tensions and prevent their accumulation? For example, you are working on a busy nursing unit staffed with one registered nurse, several students, and assistants to care for the entire patient load. This means that your assignment may be too great to accomplish adequately. You may become frustrated in carrying out the assignment, speaking sharply to the patient and your peers. You could stand around complaining about the lack of help, or you could take a few minutes to plan your work for the morning. You may not be able to give each patient the amount of time that you would like to give, but you plan to give each patient the necessary amount of care. In the latter case you are able to accomplish more for all concerned. You remain calm, the work is accomplished to the best of your ability, and good relationships are maintained. By coping effectively with your day's situation, you are better prepared to handle future situations without increasing tensions.

Alcohol. Many of you may be in the age group that is permitted to use alcohol. Socially, alcohol consumption in moderation increases interpersonal relationships between friends and acquaintances by producing a relaxed state. It may allay tensions and anxieties. Its abuse, however, is always detrimental physically and emotionally. In our rapidly changing society, alcoholism is increasing, particularly in the young. It cannot be viewed as a moral issue; it is an illness. Alcohol initially produces a feeling of well-being; latently it acts on the brain and spinal cord as a nervous system depressant. Alcoholism may lead to confusion, stupor, and mental and physical deterioration, depending on the amount and duration of consumption. Persons addicted to alcohol are seldom cured without the willpower to abstain completely from its use. One drink initiates the compulsive desire for more. Alcoholism plays an important part in crimes, accidents, the need for medical care, the breakup of families, and industrial losses from decreased production and increased absenteeism.

Smoking. It is scientifically proven that smoking has harmful physical effects by interfering with oxygen intake. Odors from smoking on the breath, hands, or clothes of the smoker may be offensive to the patient. As of January 1992 the Joint Commission on Accreditation of Hospitals has stated that all hospitals must be smoke-free or else run the risk of losing their accreditation.

Drug use. Drugs should be taken only when prescribed by and under the supervision of a physician. As a nurse you have the obligation to give only those drugs ordered by a physician. Under no condition may you make any drug available to another person without the written order of the physician.

Drug addiction is a serious problem today (see Box). It is the result of drug abuse, lack of information, "innocent" experimentation, ready availability, and the need for group identity. Scarcely a day passes that one does not read or hear about tragedies caused by drug abuse—overdoses, "bad trips," addiction, suicide, and crime. As a nurse you must not only refrain from drug abuse but also have facts and be able to recognize the common signs of abuse in others (see Table 2–1).

Commonly used addicting drugs that are available in most hospitals include narcotics such as morphine, meperidine hydrochloride (Demerol), dihydromorphinone hydrochloride (Dilaudid), and barbiturates.

Drug abuse depends on the amount and strength of the dose, the purity of the drug, and the user's surroundings, mood, emotional stability, and unique body chemistry.

Charm, Poise, and Dignity

Charm is never artificial; it is part of the person. If you are a delightful person, others want to associate with you and are pleased and happy when you come into their presence.

◆ **Behavioral Symptoms of Drug Involvement**

1. Change in work or school attendance or performance.
2. Change in personal appearance.
3. Attitude changes and mood swings.
4. Withdrawal from family contacts and responsibilities.
5. Contact with peers using drugs.
6. Strange patterns of behavior.
7. Defensive attitudes when confronted with the use of drugs.

Table 2-1 ◇ Symptoms, observations, dangers of specific drugs

Drug	Physical Symptoms	Observations	Dangers
Alcohol			
(beer, wine, liquor)	Slurred speech, unsteady walk, relaxed inhibitions, slowed reflexes, impaired coordination	Odor of alcohol on breath or clothes, hang over, drunken behavior, glazed eyes	Addiction, accidents, overdose, heart and liver damage
Cocaine			
(crack, rock, base)	Brief euphoria, elevated blood pressure and heart rate, excitement, restlessness	Possession of glass vials, pipes, white crystalline powder, syringes; needle marks on body	Addiction, seizures, lung damage, heart attack, paranoia, depression
Marijuana			
(pot, grass, hash, dope, weed, herb, joint)	Red eyes, altered perceptions, dry mouth, euphoria, reduced concentration, hunger	Odor of burnt hemp rope; possession of rolling papers, pipes, dried plant material	Addiction, impaired short-term memory, panic
Hallucinogens			
(acid, PCP, LSD, MDMA, mushrooms)	Focus on detail, anxiety, panic, nausea, altered mood and perceptions	Possession of tablets, capsules, "microdots," blotter squares	Emotional, unpredictable behavior; violent behavior (with PCP)
Inhalants			
(aerosols, gas, glue, rush, nitrites, white out)	Dizziness, nausea, headaches, lack of control and coordination	Odor of substance on clothing and breath, intoxication, poor muscular control, drowsiness	suffocation, unconsciousness nausea, vomiting, damage to central nervous system and brain, sudden death
Narcotics			
(Demerol, Dilaudid codeine,	Drowsiness, euphoria, nausea,	Possession of needles, syringes, spoons; needle marks	Addiction, lethargy, hepatitis, AIDS,

Table 2-1 ◇ *Symptoms, observations, dangers of specific drugs—cont'd*

Drug	Physical Symptoms	Observations	Dangers
Narcotics			
morphine, heroin, dope, junk, China white, black tar)	vomiting, feeling no pain, watery eyes, runny nose	on arms; pinpoint pupils; cold and moist skin	accidental overdose, weight loss
Stimulants			
(uppers, speed, Bam, crank, caffeine, black beauties crystal dexies, cocaine, nicotine	Talkativeness, alertness, wakefulness, loss of appetite, increased blood pressure, mood elevation	Loss of sleep and appetite, possession of pills and capsules, irritability or anxiety, weight loss, hyperactivity	Fatigue, addiction, paranoia, confusion, depression, possibly hallucinations
Depressants			
(barbiturates, sedatives, tranquilizers [tranks, downers, reds, ludes, Valium, yellow jackets, alcohol])	Intoxication, depressed heartbeat and breathing, drowsiness, uncoordinated movements	Confused behavior, possession of capsules and pills, longer periods of sleep, slurred speech	Possible overdose, addiction, muscle rigidity; withdrawal and overdose medical attention

Poise denotes calmness, evenness of temper, and composure. Much thought and practice are needed to obtain the desired results in this area.

Dignity implies self-control. Dignity and self-control enable you to be efficient in emergency situations and perform your designated tasks while manifesting kindness and empathy.

◆ Professionalism

As a licensed practical nurse working in a hospital or other institutional setting, you are expected to show certain types of behavior or characteristics. These include courtesy, honesty, shop talk, telephone manners, enthusiasm, and cooperation.

Courtesy

Courtesy is a polite act or remark. It is necessary in establishing satisfactory group relationships. As a nurse you must show courtesy when dealing with patients, relatives, coworkers, and other members of the health team. Courtesy is shown in many ways. A sincere, cheerful greeting ordinarily elicits a response. Its effect is contagious. Simple expressions like "thank you" and "please" produce wonders in human relationships. The most gratifying trait you can develop, if you do not already possess it, is to recognize the achievements of others through words, gestures, or actions.

You gain the cooperation of your patient by being courteous to him. Indicate that you respect him by addressing him properly, using his correct name, "Mr. Smith." Refrain from calling him "Pop" or "Grandpa" or by his first name. Every patient wants to retain his identity. Another courteous gesture is explaining in advance any procedure you must perform in terms the patient understands. This explanation alleviates anxiety and indicates that you care about the patient as a person.

One important form of courtesy you must remember as a nurse is to knock on a closed door before entering. This may save the patient embarrassment and secures the right to privacy. Other forms of politeness include not interrupting a conversation unless absolutely necessary, stepping aside to allow someone in a hurry to pass easily, offering an apology, and excusing yourself when leaving a group.

Honesty

A practical nurse must be a person of high integrity. The nursing profession trusts you to act in the best interests of the patient. This includes charting treatments and medications accurately, carrying out physicians' orders as written, reporting errors immediately to the proper authorities, not willfully performing or assisting with any procedure or act detrimental to the patient, and performing only those procedures for which you have been sufficiently prepared and are within the scope of the Nurse Practice Act.

Honesty and economy work hand in hand. If you are honest with your employer and your patients, you will not waste time or materials. Wastefulness is costly and may result in an increase in hospital operating expenses. Ultimately this cost is reflected in the patient's bill. Time is a costly item to all institutions and businesses. When added together, minutes spent daydreaming, talking about others, and avoiding work amount to large sums of wasted money. Lost time lowers the standards of nursing care.

Careless use of equipment and materials is costly to the patient and the hospital. Because of their delicacy and unique craftsmanship, hospital equipment and supplies are expensive items. Thoughtless contamination of sterile equipment may cause harm to your patient and result in infectious processes and financial deficits. Learn to use time, equipment, and supplies to the best possible advantage.

Shop Talk

Shop talk is common among employees. It may be defined as a discussion of the various factors of one's work. There is no harm in discussing work itself. However, when it involves names, personalities, and a physician's treatment of a patient, it is unethical. Do not become too personal. Talk about general things. Do not discuss work in public places. Avoid gossiping about other personnel; it is disloyal and unfair. Take great care in answering questions of relatives, patients, and members of the health care team.

Telephone Manners

The telephone is an important means of communication (see the box below).

Hospital telephones are limited to professional calls. Personal calls are referred to the personnel or nursing service departments or to the nursing school office. In case of emergency these departments take a message and deliver it to you, or they transfer the call directly to you.

Enthusiasm and Cooperation

Enthusiasm and cooperation are treasured characteristics. They help build employee morale and create good working conditions and relationships between departments within the institution. They stimulate workers to give their best to the job.

Enthusiasm should never encroach on the duties of fellow workers. Never attempt to assume anyone else's duties. Most institutions have job descriptions stating the specific duties for each job category. Job descriptions define and eliminate overlapping activities among employees. Enthusiasm and cooperation imply helping others and working together with a genuine interest in what each is accomplishing for the patient's welfare. Enthusiasm and cooperation make the patient feel secure and confident. They assure the patient that all are interested in his recovery and are willing to do whatever is necessary and requested.

Professional Patient-Nurse Communication

What is the patient's reaction to you, the nurse? What is the patient's role in the hospital? Patients are ill persons who have been transported from their own environment to an entirely new environment to which they must adjust. The patient identifies the hospital and each member of the health team as one. Ordinarily the patient does not make a distinction between the registered nurse, the practical nurse, the nursing

---

◆ **Rules for Telephone Use**

1. Answer in a friendly tone of voice and be courteous.
2. Identify your location, name, and title.
3. Summon the proper person to the phone or record the message.
4. All calls made on duty should be brief, courteous, accurate, and necessary.
5. Never give unauthorized information over the phone. Always know to whom you are speaking.
6. When receiving a call that requires time to gather the needed information, ask the caller to hold or ask to return the call. Make sure you have the correct number if you are to return the call.
7. Replace the receiver gently.

assistant, the x-ray technician, or any other member of the health care team. Patients regard the ones caring for them as the persons directly responsible for their immediate care and recovery. Patients watch your every move, your responses to their illness and the symptoms it manifests, and your actions and dealings with other patients. Patients judge you in view of these actions to assure themselves that they are in capable hands and will recover through your efficient, kind, and conscientious care.

Patients are also fearful. The hospital setting may be foreign to them. Patients do not know what is expected of them in the hospital's daily routine. You allay some of these fears if you take time to explain things the patient needs to know. For example, you may tell the patient to go "down the hall" to take a shower. "Down the hall" to the patient may mean going to another nursing division, which may be a distance down the hall, or it may mean several doors from the room. It is simpler to say, "Mrs. Jones, the bathroom or shower is five doors down the corridor on the right hand side." This short explanation clearly describes the location of the bathroom and allays the patient's anxiety and fear of the unknown. It is easy for you to take things for granted, especially after you have become acquainted with the hospital setting. It becomes a second home to you, but when you started as a new student, you were often frustrated. Your instructors helped you to overcome this frustration, but who is to help the patient?

As a student practical nurse, you spend much time at the bedside. You have the opportunity to become acquainted with the patient and to explain details to the patient that are often taken for granted and assumed that the patient knows. Be empathetic to the patient. Empathy is an attempt to experience the individual's emotional state as if you were in the individual's place. It allows the patient's world to become the nurse's world for a time. Such involvement helps the nurse to see patients as they are and not as they "ought" to be. It helps the nurse to become more appreciative of the feelings of others.

The nurse must establish a personalized communication with the patient. This is difficult to do with someone you do not know or if there is a difference in age, sex, race, or culture. Persons usually interpret what is communicated according to their customary ways of thinking and their patterns of experience. In these matters the nurse must remain objective to prevent personal values from changing the meaning of the message. The patient has been taken from the home situation and placed in the hospital setting. The patient knows exactly where everything is at home but not in the hospital. The patient may watch favorite television programs routinely but may not even have a television in the room. The patient may be in a double room with a person who appears very ill and whom the patient believes may die. The patient immediately begins to think, "I wonder if they'll find that I have something serious and that I may die." The other patient may not be acutely ill or dying but merely appears so to the new patient. The two may remain strangers to each other because no one has introduced them. When you entered nursing school, you may have had to introduce yourself to your companions, and this may have been difficult for you. Perhaps you even shied away from others, and then you were lonely. A patient frequently experiences these same problems when admitted to a hospital, but problems are minimized if hospital personnel are friendly and the nurse takes the time to explain things and establish a rapport with the patient.

A patient must endure various restrictions when in a hospital. For example, at home friends visit as often and as long as they desire. In a hospital, certain hours are set aside for visiting. At times visitors may not be treated in as friendly a manner as the patient wishes them to be treated, and this causes the patient to feel hurt and uncomfortable. The following are examples of unfriendly treatment of visitors:

1. You enter the room to perform some particular patient procedure and find that the patient has visitors. Because you are hurried as a result of having much to do, you appear curt and say as few words as possible, such as "Please leave the room."
2. On entering the room and finding the patient has visitors, you turn around and walk out without saying a word.

Neither patients nor their visitors would object if you were to ask the visitors in a pleasant voice to wait in the hall or in the waiting room for a few minutes. You could simply explain that you wish to perform some procedure for the patient. If possible, you could also say, "Hello, Mr. Jones, I see that you have visitors. I have a procedure to do that can wait; I'll return when visiting hours are over." This approach allows the patient and visitors to feel comfortable with you. They feel accepted by you and are more willing to cooperate with you. A few words and gestures make a great deal of difference. If you were in a fellow student's room and another student walked in suddenly, saw you, and left immediately without saying anything, you would feel uncomfortable. The patient experiences these same feelings.

Patients are knowledgeable consumers. They are aware of the cost of a hospital and expect services equal to that cost. The hospital and personnel are often judged by the quality of care rendered. Therefore it is important that the patient be made to feel secure and safe and to know that care will be given in a concerned and empathetic manner (see the box on p. 22). Hospital personnel are "ambassadors of good will." Their behavior and the care they administer often enhance or negate the reputation of a health care facility.

The Hospital

The hospital may be large or small. Regardless of size, it is simply a structure filled with many skilled people, ranging from the administrator of the hospital to the janitor. It consists of various departments, each with a specific purpose. Each department affects the patient and you, either directly or indirectly. If one department fails to do an efficient job, everyone feels the effects of this failure. The hospital contains large quantities of different types of equipment. Each has its specific function, and it may benefit you to learn as much as you can about it.

The hospital has rules and regulations that are made to ensure order and uniformity, to safeguard the institution, and to provide the best care for the patient. For example, a physician knows that early ambulation is necessary to promote a full range of motion and healing. If the nurse decides that this order is severe and ambulates the patient only once a day, this decision may have serious consequences for the patient. It may necessitate a repeat operation, a prolonged hospital stay, or failure of complete recovery without full range of motion. The patient needs to be assured that all personnel are working for his improvement and that orders written by the physician are being carried out accurately. The physician, who has the full responsibility for the medical care

---

◆ Patient Rights and Responsibilities

1. In recognition of their human dignity, all patients have a right to considerate and respectful quality medical care rendered by competent personnel.
2. All patients have the right to obtain from their physician current information concerning diagnosis, treatment, and prognosis in terms the patient can understand. Patients have the responsibility to cooperate in their treatment program.
3. All patients have the right to be informed and choose alternative treatments including the right to refuse treatment to the extent permitted by law. Patients are responsible for their own actions if they refuse treatment.
4. All patients have the right to privacy concerning their medical care.
5. All patients have the right to expect the hospital to make a reasonable response to their request for services.
6. All patients have the right to expect reasonable continuity of care and assistance in locating alternate services when medically indicated.
7. All patients have the right to examine and receive an explanation of their bill. Patients have the responsibility to provide information necessary for claim processing and to be prompt in payment of bills.
8. Patients are entitled to information about the mechanism for the initiation, review, and resolution of patient complaints.
9. Patients are responsible for being considerate of the rights of other patients and personnel, and for assisting in the control of noise, smoking, and the number of visitors.

Courtesy St. Mary's Health Center, St Louis, Missouri

---

of the patient, works within the framework of the hospital and abides by its rules and regulations. As previously stated, the registered nurse has the responsibility for the direct nursing care of the patient. The practical nurse works under the supervision of the registered nurse and administers patient care. Both are directly responsible to their employer and are obligated to follow the policies of the hospital.

The patient's care is planned to ensure the uniformity vital to recovery. The nursing care plan is a written, individualized course of action to meet the total needs of the patient. This specified method assists the patient to adjust physically and emotionally. The following example helps to clarify the need for this written, individualized plan of action. A patient has a leg amputated and after full recovery has a prosthesis attached. On Monday a nurse enters the room and states, "I'm sorry your leg had to be amputated, Mr. Jones. I'll give you a bath to make it easier for you." In this instance the nurse expresses pity for the patient and makes the patient dependent. This is a poor approach because it delays the patient's progress and recovery by encouraging dependency. On Tuesday morning another nurse enters the room and remarks, "Mr. Jones, it's time for your morning bath. I'll bring you some warm water so that you can bathe yourself. I know that you can do this, but if you have any difficulty, I'll be glad to help you." At this point Mr. Jones must be thinking, "One nurse wants to do everything for me, whereas the second nurse wants me to do everything for myself. I wish they would get together so that I would know what they want me to do. One nurse feels sorry for me, but the other nurse accepts my condition." If Mr. Jones has a tendency to feel sorry for himself, he will dislike the second nurse, who failed to indulge him. The second nurse, however, is aware that the patient needs to accept his condition and help himself. A careful assessment and a well-written nursing care plan help eliminate this type of situation because the plan states a definite approach to be used by all nursing personnel.

A hospital team (doctors, nurses, technicians, dietitians, social workers, therapists, and others) must work together toward a common goal if that goal is to be attained. A team whose spirit is high accomplishes much; a team whose spirit is low accomplishes little. The patient suffers as a result of poor team spirit.

In summary the practical nurse is a caring, educated individual practicing within the parameters and scope of the Nurse Practice Act. The practical nurse is well groomed, well mannered, cheerful, honest, responsible, and respected. The practical nurse knows and respects the rights of the patient, renders quality and professional care, and adheres to the rules and regulations of the institution.

Bibliography

Bernhard LA, Walsh M: *Leadership,* ed 2, St Louis, 1990, Mosby.
Chenevert M: *Mosby's tour guide to nursing school,* ed 2, St Louis, 1992, Mosby.
McCloskey JC, Grace HK: *Current issues in nursing,* ed 3, St Louis, 1990, Mosby.
Williams SJ, Guerra SJ: *Health care services in the 1990s,* ed 1, New York, 1991, Praeger.

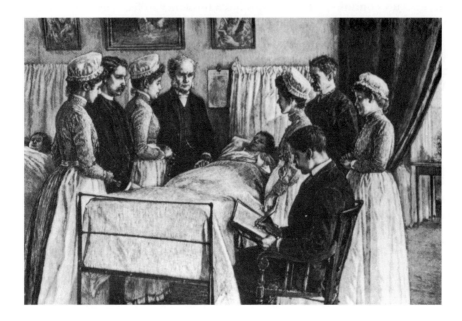

Objectives

At the completion of this chapter the student practical nurse will be able to:

◆ Describe the development of nursing from ancient times to modern day.

◆ Describe the development of practical nursing from its earliest time through the modern day.

◆ Identify by name and accomplishment those who influenced nursing and practical nursing.

◆ Explain the role of the practical nurse as a member of the health team.

3 History and Trends of Professional and Practical Nursing

When you think of history, your thoughts often revert to something that is ancient and dead. However, history is in the making every day. Your actions today in some way affect the lives of others tomorrow. They serve to pave the road of the nursing profession to greater achievements. Because your actions and activities have far-reaching effects on the future, you should know the part the past has played in your life today. Nursing dates back to the earliest times of mankind.

◆ Nursing in Ancient Civilizations

In ancient times nursing was not a formal occupation based on scientific principles. The development of nursing in history is closely linked with, although not necessarily parallel to, medical history. It is probable that neither medicine nor nursing could have developed without the other. Nursing existed in practice although not in name.

Nursing functions were frequently performed by a member of a sick person's household, a relative, or a servant. Childbirth was accompanied by some type of nursing care of mother and child by midwives and wet nurses. The temple, a center of religion, was a healing place where nursing functions were performed by a priest, priestess, or deaconess.

As medicine developed scientifically, physicians began to impart their knowledge to students, who were responsible for the care and observation of the patient.

With advancement of the woman's position in society and achievement of educational, economic, and political freedoms, parallel gains were made in nursing. This freedom for women was necessary for nursing to develop as a profession.

Babylonia

In early Mesopotamia, sickness was regarded as a punishment for sin, and the ill were cared for within the household by a slave or domestic servant. Historical documents prove that nursing duties such as bathing, bandaging, and massaging the patient were performed in this civilization.

One of the ancient Babylonian kings, Hammurabi, compiled a code of law (2000 BC) that placed legal limitations on those treating the sick. This code was designed as a protective measure for patients.

Egypt

Egyptian medicine contained contrasting elements of mysticism, realism, magic, and empiricism.

Training schools for physicians were attached to many of the temples. There is evidence that one such school existed around 1100 BC. Temple priests were responsible for nursing care functions such as bathing. Medical students were involved in the care and observation of patients. In addition, lay persons with special knowledge or talents in this area were frequently excused from work to care for the sick.

The best source of knowledge about ancient Egyptian nursing techniques is found in the *Edwin Smith Surgical Papyrus,* which gives detailed instructions for the daily care of patients.

It may surprise today's nurses to know that their counterparts in ancient Egypt recorded the pulse and used present-day techniques and materials, such as bandages and splints, in the care and treatment of the sick and wounded.

Israel

The Old Testament is an excellent resource on Hebrew history. Many passages refer to wet nurses and those who nursed the sick or acted as companions.*

In the area of medicine the Hebrew priest functioned as a public health officer. Nursing, confined to the home, was rendered by women of the community.

Although the Hebrews borrowed their medical knowledge from the Babylonians and Egyptians, they were unique in that they generously shared this knowledge with succeeding civilizations.

Greece

The Greek woman's lack of freedom limited the progress of nursing because it restricted nursing duties to household members.

However, progress in the field of medicine was monumental and indirectly affected nursing. Hippocrates (460–370 BC) was responsible for this medical progress. He introduced the scientific method in the diagnosis and treatment of patients, which eliminated the mythical and magical elements of treatment. For 2000 years Hippocrates has been known as the Father of Medicine.

His emphasis on close observation, medical and surgical treatment, and care of patients reveals a dependence of physicians on medical students and trained nurses to carry out these functions. The Greeks were the first to become conscious of the need for *trained* nurses.

In Greek society, birth was also attended by midwives and nurses. Socrates' mother was a nurse-midwife.

---

*Numbers 11:12; Exodus 2:7, 2:9; II Kings 4:4; Genesis 24:59, 35:8.

Rome

Roman medicine was a product of that civilization's thirst for conquest. Greek physicians who were Roman prisoners of war brought with them Hippocratic medicine. Before this time medicine was a mixture of common sense remedies and superstition.

Although the Romans added little to the field of medicine, they recognized the need for nursing and expanded it into a specialized field. Their conquests were responsible for the establishment of military hospitals with nurse attendants. Roman soldiers were trained in basic first aid techniques. Buildings or rooms on large Roman estates served as hospitals and were staffed by "professional nurses" who were probably slaves.

China

There is no reference in the literature of Ancient China to nurses. If there were nurses, they probably were not women, because Confucius defined woman's position as inferior to man. The woman's place was in the home, and her greatest value was when she produced a son.

India

Ancient Indian writings from 800 BC to 2 AD set standards and qualifications for male nurses. These included knowledge, preparation and compounding of drugs for administration, devotedness to the patient, cleverness, and purity of body and mind. Technical skills, which included bathing, rubbing and massaging, lifting and moving the patient, and bedmaking, were emphasized. Nurses were to be untiring in their service to the sick.

◆ Nursing in the Early Christian Era (50–476 AD)

About the time of Christ's birth, Rome had reached its supremacy. Christianity was rarely manifested openly because it was prohibited by the emperor. However, as Rome declined, Christianity spread and grew. Organized nursing came into existence as an expression of charity. St. Paul introduced Phoebe of Cenchreae into Rome as a deaconess of the church. One of her duties was to care for the sick. Phoebe is known as the first visiting nurse and the first deaconess in the church. Grasping the spirit of this new Christianity, other Christian convents formed orders to care for the sick and poor.

History records that Fabiola, a wealthy matron, founded a hospital in Rome in atonement for the sin of having a second marriage. She rendered personal care to the sick and injured, and no disease was too grave or too contagious to prevent her from giving care. Her good deeds became known among the elite. In a short time Marcella and Paula, two other wealthy matrons, joined in this charitable work. Nursing progressed until the Dark Ages.

◆ Nursing in the Dark Ages (476–1000 AD)

Little is known about nursing in the Dark Ages. However, we know that learning of all types was kept alive through the great literary works of that period. Christians, who brought about organized nursing care, were again persecuted, and followers of Christianity hid behind walls of monasteries and convents. Various religions included in their practices not only the conversion of heathens but also the care of the sick. In the medical field, hospitals were founded. The most noted were Hôtel-Dieu in Lyons in 542 AD, Hôtel-Dieu in Paris in 650 AD, and Santo Spirito in Rome in 717 AD. Although nursing history during this period remains obscure, it is assumed, because new hospitals were founded and staffed by trained personnel who enabled the hospitals to achieve the fame for which they are known and recorded in history.

◆ Nursing in the Middle Ages (1000–1450 AD)

The two main factors influencing nursing during the Middle Ages were religion and the military. Because monks and nuns assumed most of the nursing duties, new and additional monasterial orders were founded. A number of these were military orders that trained men in the techniques of fighting and the care of the sick. One such order was the Knights Hospitalers, who were formally approved by the pope in 1113. Men belonging to this order ministered to their own sick and wounded soldiers. They worked in general hospitals rendering the needed nursing care and fought in defense of the reigning political power. Two additional military orders, the Knights Templars and Teutonic Knights, came into existence. All performed similar duties and received uniform training. As time progressed, the religious duty of caring for the sick predominated over the military duty. This is not surprising in view of the fact that the primary concern of established religious orders was the care of the sick and poor.

During the Middle Ages cleanliness and ventilation as known today were nonexistent. Buildings were constructed with windows too high to open. There were few, if any, facilities for plumbing, heating, and lighting. In many instances linens had to be carried to and washed in the river. Nursing care was primitive and consisted chiefly of administering medications, bathing patients, dressing wounds, and providing for the physical needs of patients.

Accustomed as we are in the United States to the latest conveniences in hospital construction, facilities, and equipment, we would consider medical facilities and nursing care in the Middle Ages crude and deficient. However, similar conditions exist today in poverty-stricken and underdeveloped nations. In these countries, hospitals are constructed without heat, with poor lighting with frequently nonfunctioning electric power, and with inadequate plumbing to meet patients' needs. Linens are washed in cold water in outdoor concrete sinks and are cleansed by rubbing soiled areas with rough rocks. Inhabitants of such countries wash their clothing in nearby streams and rivers. Nursing remains primitive. Medications are given to the patient only if the family provides them. Bathing is infrequent because of lack of heat and warm water. The nurse dresses wounds, assists with uncomplicated surgical procedures (complicated procedures are not performed), and attempts to meet the physical needs of patients. Are these not conditions similar to those that existed in the Middle Ages?

During the Middle Ages, societal structure changed to include a third, or middle, class of people between the poor and the rich. Several factors united and effected this development. The Christian religion dominated all aspects of the Western world. The church functioned as the head and power of the collective small cities in Europe. Cathedrals and universities were founded. Buying and selling between cities and, later, nations became a common practice. The cultural flow between Europe and the Orient was initiated by those participating in the Crusades. The combination of these factors necessitated the development of a middle class to carry forward these achievements.

Nursing was also affected by the development of the middle class. This is illustrated by the life and activities of St. Catherine of Siena (1347–1380). Catherine gave herself untiringly to the care of the sick. When the plague came to Siena in 1372, she worked day and night nursing its victims. The greatest problem at this time was the need for some type of transportation of the sick to hospitals. In response to this need, Catherine organized the first ambulance service. Today the Hospital at La Scala stands as a memorial to Catherine for her heroic efforts and accomplishments during this period.

Near the close of the Middle Ages the church had lost much of its power, and monastic life no longer attracted young people. Therefore fewer persons were dedicated to the care of the sick. Several new orders were formed; one was the Beguines of Flanders, founded in 1184. This order devoted itself to the service of the sick and poor but functioned independently of church authority. As a result of the decreased number of practitioners, a great demand was created in the nursing field.

◆ The Decline of Nursing: Nursing from the Renaissance to the Nineteenth Century (1450–1800)

Although during the Renaissance, Protestants urged the state to accept responsibility for the care of the sick, Catholics tried to salvage some of their nursing orders. At this time there were no experienced nurses to care for the ill except those within religious orders.

Because state officials showed little concern for hospitals established for the poor, hospitals and nursing care declined rapidly. It seems apparent that no sense of charity existed among the rich. When plague afflicted the people, the rich fled from the cities, leaving the poor without proper medication, food, and care. However, this period was not without magnanimous persons. John Howard (1727–1789), Mother Mary Catherine McAuley (1787–1841), and William Tuke (1732–1822) recognized the disastrous situation and attempted to reform nursing care and conditions in hospitals, prisons, and mental institutions. One of the outstanding men of this era, St. Vincent de Paul, dedicated his life as a priest to improving conditions for the sick. In 1600 he founded the Order of the Sisters of Charity with the assistance of Louise de Marillac. This order exists today, and its members continue to devote their time and efforts to the care of the poor and sick.

◆ The Beginning of Modern Nursing

Nursing Before Florence Nightingale

By the end of the eighteenth century, nursing had reached its lowest ebb in Protestant countries. Educated women of the upper class disapproved of manual labor and no longer cared for the sick and needy. It was considered a disgrace to send a member of the family to the hospital; therefore the sick were cared for in the home. Charles Dickens' novel *Martin Chuzzlewit* (1844), with its Sairey Gamp and Betsey Prig, best portrays nurses of this time as being women of immoral standards who were unsympathetic, alcohol-imbibing, and unfeeling individuals.

In Catholic communities in America the nursing situation was less devastating because priests and nuns who arrived with French and Spanish settlers possessed small amounts of nursing knowledge and skills. In Latin American countries nursing care was given by Catholic nursing orders. Hospitals existed in other countries long before they were established in the United States. The most commonly known orders in both North and South American hospitals were the Augustinian nuns, Ursuline nuns, and Sisters of Charity.

The first established school of nursing was founded in Kaiserswerth, Germany, in 1836 by a German pastor, Theodor Fliedner, who founded a hospital in his parish. With the assistance of an experienced nurse, Gertrude Reichardt, he revived the practice of deaconesses performing nursing functions. After 1 to 3 years of theory and practice the graduates of Kaiserswerth Deaconess Institution traveled to other parts of the world and founded similar programs. Florence Nightingale received her training at Kaiserswerth. Modern nursing begins with the Florence Nightingale era.

Nursing During the Florence Nightingale Era (1820–1910)

Florence Nightingale not only was the founder of modern nursing but also made it the respected career it is today. She was born of a wealthy family in Florence, Italy, on May 12, 1820. The year after her birth, Florence's family returned to England, and it was there she received her education. Despite her elite learning, social graces, and family opposition, Florence Nightingale was possessed by a need to care for the sick and entered Kaiserswerth Deaconess Institution in 1851 to study nursing. She later worked and studied with the Sisters of Charity in Paris.

The first position held by Nightingale was that of superintendent of a small institution in London, the Establishment for Gentlewomen During Illness. She worked diligently planning nursing care for her patients, and her efforts were rewarded. She was happy and successful. Nightingale strongly advocated that nursing existed for the healthy and for the sick.

When the Crimean War broke out, Russia and France had religious sisters to care for their wounded and sick, but England had only untrained men. Florence Nightingale eagerly answered the call for help that came to her from the Secretary of War. On October 21, 1854, she set out with her small chosen group of nurses to serve her country and humanity.

In caring for the wounded soldiers, Florence Nightingale met and tackled obstacles of filth, poor diet, understaffing, and inefficiency. She saw these deplorable conditions as a challenge and used her administrative genius in selecting nurses, erecting hospitals, and initiating much needed reforms. She provided the soldiers with clean bedding, nourishing food, hospital clothing, and skilled nurses to care for them. For her efforts she was honored with the title of Lady of the Lamp. Through her work during the war she broke down the age-old prejudice of the world toward nursing.

In 1862 William Rathbone begged Nightingale to assist him in establishing a home nursing service in London. Her response to this plea was the establishment of the Training School and Home for Nurses of the Royal Infirmary. This program provided nurses for private duty, the hospital, and the district. This project marked the beginning of modern visiting nursing, better known today as *public health nursing.*

Florence Nightingale opened up the field of nursing as a profession. She was influential in establishing improved nursing programs and schools of nursing, improving woman's place in society and in the military, raising the standards of hospitals and facilities, and initiating the philosophy of "treating the patient rather than the disease." Florence served as the world's advisor on hospital matters and nursing service. She wrote many books; among her best known are *Notes on Nursing* and *Notes on Hospitals,* both published in 1859.

Florence Nightingale died in 1910 at age 90. Although she suffered criticisms and endured trials in order to succeed, her courage and stamina will be remembered forever. She saw nursing as a necessity and a challenge and fought for it. Her efforts were not in vain. Today nursing is the profession she wanted it to be.

Another outstanding nurse of the Florence Nightingale era was Ella King Newsom. Newsom was Nightingale's counterpart with the American Confederate Army. Newsom received her training at Memphis City Hospital from the Sisters of Mercy and the medical staff. She applied her unusual organizational and executive abilities to erecting and administering hospitals while following the retreating Confederate Army. Her hospitals were noted for their cleanliness and humane treatment of the wounded.

◆ Nursing in the Late Nineteenth and Early Twentieth Centuries (1890–1960)

The greatest developments in modern nursing occurred during and after the Nightingale era, and nursing owes much to the leaders of this time. It was through their interest and tireless efforts that nursing advanced from an apprenticeship to a profession. It is difficult to read of the activities of these leaders without being caught up in the spirit that inspired and energized these dedicated persons.

Jean H. Dunant, a Swiss, formulated a plan of international relief for the masses of victims of war and calamity. The plan provided for independent associations and societies for war relief in each country with a strong international bond of affiliation among countries and a guaranteed neutrality of supplies and personnel. The plan was agreed on by representatives of 16 nations at the Geneva Conference in Switzerland in 1863. This agreement led to the formation of the International Red Cross Society. The society proposed to prepare in advance for war and disaster by gathering and storing all needed equipment such as medical and surgical supplies, clothing, portable shelters, furniture, and tools in large warehouses.

Because of the Civil War the United States was not present at the Geneva Conference and was the thirty-second country to enter the International Red Cross; thus the need to form a similar society in the United States, the American Red Cross Society, was recognized. This was accomplished through the tireless efforts of Clara Barton, a nurse in the Civil War. She organized the Red Cross Committee in Washington, based on Nightingale customs and persuaded government officials to give the committee official standing in 1882. Clara Barton was the first president of the American Red Cross.

The Red Cross Society in the United States has given and loaned money and supplies to devastated areas and has helped rebuild houses or reestablish businesses. Outside the United States the organization has given supplies and aid in the reconstruction of countries where volcanic eruptions, floods, epidemics, and other disasters have occurred.

During this period medicine and nursing were making revolutionary strides. Louis Pasteur and Robert Koch introduced scientific discoveries and medical treatment based on bacteriologic studies. Joseph Lister developed surgical antiseptic techniques that helped decrease the number of wound infections and deaths after surgical procedures. The process of nursing followed that of medicine, with a number of outstanding women giving greater dimension to the new profession.

Dorothea Dix, a retired schoolteacher, was a strong promoter of improving conditions and treatment of the mentally ill. Her first contact with the mentally ill was in a jail in East Cambridge, Massachusetts, in 1841. She was appalled at the environmental conditions existing in the jail where many mentally ill prisoners were held. Treatment of the prisoners ranged from indifference to brutality. She obtained data, secured the support of influential citizens, and presented these facts to government officials and to courts of law. Her efforts brought about improvements in jails and the establishment of psychiatric institutions.

To improve poor conditions existing in military camps, which included lack of care for sick soldiers and inadequacies of supplies, drugs, and transportation, Dorothea Dix was appointed Superintendent of the Female Nurses of the Army in 1861. Without military rank or a background of nurse's training, Dix organized military hospitals, obtained needed materials, and supplied nurses to comfort and minister to the wounded and sick soldiers.

Linda Richards, the first trained nurse in America, graduated from the New England Hospital for Women and Children in Boston in 1872. After graduation her first assignment was night superintendent at Bellevue. One year later she was appointed superintendent of the Boston Training School. In addition to her teaching duties, she gave patient care and devoted long hours to the care of the sick. As a medical missionary in Japan from 1885 to 1889, Richards established and directed the first training school for nurses in that country. Her remaining efforts were devoted to establishing nursing schools in hospitals for the mentally ill.

Near the turn of the century Isabel Hampton Robb (1860–1910) was linked with every type of organization, plan, and activity in nursing. She was a constructive thinker who applied her ideas practically. In 1889 she initiated important reforms in nursing such as policies for a 12-hour day for student nurses; time allowance for meals, rest, study, and recreation periods; and a maximum limit to the workday. She helped eliminate private duty as part of the student nurse's education. In 1895 she advocated an 8-hour day for student nurses, the termination of stipends to raise the student nurse from the position of employee to that of student, and a 3-year nurse training program. She believed that licensing examinations and registration would protect patients from incompetent nurses and raise the status and standards of nurses. She was the first president of the Nurses Associated Alumnae of the United States and Canada, the first principal of the Johns Hopkins School of Nursing, and one of the founders and original stockholders of the *American Journal of Nursing*.

Mary Adelaide Nutting (1858–1947) was a graduate of the first class at the Johns Hopkins School of Nursing and a friend of Isabel Hampton Robb. She continued the reforms initiated by Robb.

Her many accomplishments include separation of nursing schools from hospital ownership through state support for schools of nursing, raising the educational standards of basic nursing programs, founding nursing organizations, and creating and developing the Department of Nursing and Health at Teacher's College, Columbia University. She was honored with the title of First Professor of Nursing and was influential in the formation of the International Council of Nurses. In 1944 the National League of Nursing Education awarded Nutting the first medal for leadership, the Adelaide Nutting Medal for Leadership in Nursing Education.

Lillian Wald (1867–1940) is best known as the foundress of the famed Henry Street Settlement. This event in 1893 marked the beginning of the development of the social service aspects of nursing as well as modern nursing in the community. The Henry Street Settlement, which began in a top-floor tenement on the Lower East Side of New York City, was established as a neighborhood nursing service for the sick poor. Wald's intensive crusade to assist the poor was based on her desire to nurse the poor as a friend rather than as a paid visitor. This was the true beginning of public health nursing in the United States.

Annie Goodrich (1876–1955) was the instigator of the Army School of Nursing in 1918. This school was founded as a war measure but was designed to continue as a permanent organization. The 3-year course granted 9 months of credit to college graduates entering the program. The students' work was centered in army hospitals, and in 1920 officer's rank was granted to nurses.

In addition to Goodrich's endeavors in the Army School of Nursing, she was president of the International Council of Nurses from 1912 to 1915, Director of the Visiting Nurse Service of the Henry Street Settlement in 1916, and Dean of Nursing at Yale.

Nutting, Wald, and Goodrich are frequently referred to as The Great Trio in the rapid development of nursing during this period.

Mary E. Mahoney, America's first black graduate nurse, pressed for integration, better working conditions, and health care facilities in the Boston area. This pioneering nurse formed the National Association for Colored Graduate Nurses (NACGN).

In her doctoral thesis, "Education of nursing technicians," Mildred L. Montag proposed the establishment of a new position above the level of the practical nurse and below the level of the professional nurse. This position has been made possible by programs offered by the junior and community colleges. It is the Associate Degree of Nursing (ADN). These programs are scattered throughout the United States.

Another important person in nursing history is Isabel Maitland Stewart (1878–1963). Stewart was influential in upgrading the educational status of nursing and in changing the thinking of nursing leaders in the United States and abroad. She was the first nurse to receive a master's degree from Columbia University.

These dedicated nursing pioneers were totally involved in all aspects of nursing: military, international, educational, social, and public health. They were active in nursing organizations, reforms, and improvements. Their legacy to us is found in their numerous writings.

Today nursing patterns are changing rapidly. Domestic tasks are no longer included in the duties of the registered nurse, who is assuming greater responsibility for the supervision of personnel, complicated medical and surgical procedures, and planning and implementing patient care in hospitals, homes, and community projects. The nurse is functioning in a leadership role. Nursing is now worldwide.

Space exploration has opened a new field for nurses. At the present this means caring for astronauts and their families, but in the future the nurse's role will expand to include numerous other facets in the aerospace program.

◆ Practical Nursing

The practical nurse became a permanent member of the health care team when society needed a trained person who could render competent and intelligent bedside care to patients. The need for a training program for practical nurses was recognized early, and in 1893 the first school for practical nurses in the United States, the Ballard School, which consisted of a 3-month program, was founded in New York. Two other forerunners of the practical nursing schools of today were the Thompson School, founded in Brattleboro, Vermont, in 1907, and the Household Nursing Association School of Attendant Nursing, established in 1918 in Boston for the purpose of training practical nurses to give care in the home.

The Household Nursing Association School, the name of which was changed to Shepard-Gill School of Practical Nursing, closed in 1985. In our present system practical nursing programs are offered by hospitals, vocational-technical schools, and junior and community colleges.

In 1941, 28 people met in Chicago and formed the Association of Practical Nurse Schools. Hilda M. Torrop, Director of the Ballard School; Etta Creech, Director of the Family Health Association in Cleveland; and Katherine Shepard, Executive Director of the Household Nursing Association in Boston, were founders and officers of the association. Hilda Torrop later became the first executive director. In 1942 membership was opened to practical nurses, and the name of the association was changed to the National Association for Practical Nurse Education (NAPNE). In 1945 NAPNE established an accrediting service for practical nursing schools. It began holding a summer school and workshops for directors and instructors in 1950. And in 1951 it started the first practical nursing magazine, now called the *Journal of Practical Nursing*. By 1953 it was sponsoring summer continuing education programs for practical nurses. As time passed, the continuing education and welfare of practical nurses received more and more emphasis. In 1959 a Department of Service to State Practical Nursing Associations and a Department of Education were established, and the name of the association was changed to the National Association for Practical Nurse Education and Services (NAPNES).

In 1949 the National Federation of Licensed Practical Nurses (NFLPN) was organized by Lillian Kuster as the official membership organization for licensed practical nurses. Through the efforts of NAPNES and NFLPN the general public became aware of practical nursing, its educational programs, and the licensure of practical nurses. In 1955 all the states passed licensure laws affecting practical nursing.

In 1957 the Council on Practical Nursing (now Council of Practical Nursing Programs) was established under the auspices of the National League for Nursing (NLN) to help establish and maintain high-quality programs in schools of practical nursing. And in 1961 it became a department within the Division of Nursing Education. In 1962 the NFLPN founded the National Licensed Practical Nurses Educational Foundation for research, development of continuing education programs, and the awarding of scholarships to licensed practical nurses. It was through the combined efforts of NAPNES, NFLPN, and NLN that practical nursing became an integral part of nursing.

In 1979 the National League for Nursing councils developed, adopted, and published competencies of graduates of educational programs in practical nursing. Today practical nursing students are prepared by qualified nurse educators in structured health care settings such as hospitals. Clinical practice is correlated with basic therapeutic knowledge, mental health concepts, biologic and behavioral sciences, and communication skills. Planned and supervised experiences are directed toward teaching students using current concepts and practices.

With the changes in the 1980s and 1990s, practical nurses are facing added responsibilities every day. The practical nurse now must assume more duties than ever before and make decisions during crises. We are in a time of rapid change that will continue.

In hospitals throughout the United States practical nurses make up a vital part of the organizational structure. Professional nurses are unable to function adequately without the assistance of practical nurses because of increased patient acuity, advances in technology, complexity of nursing care, and the demands of society. The function of the practical nurse is to render personalized bedside patient care and assist with care in complex situations. On successful completion of courses in an approved school, the practical nurse may function in the capacity of medicine nurse, team leader, or charge nurse. Completion of additional courses prepares the practical nurse for intravenous therapy.

Practical nurse programs do not prepare the nurse to go on to professional nursing, but in 1968 the NLN Council of Diploma Programs passed a resolution to make every effort to admit the licensed practical nurse (LPN) to diploma programs. This allows the LPN to challenge by examination those materials already learned and to move from one level of nursing to another with more ease. Since 1970 a greater effort has been made to allow LPNs to challenge course work through competency-based modules.

Some ADN programs offer a transition program after a specified amount of practical experience has been gained. Other schools have a ladder program in which the student stops after the first year and takes the LPN examination or continues for the second year and takes the RN examination.

In rural areas students may want to check on approved External Degree Programs (correspondence courses with periodic testing at selected sites). This may be an easier and less expensive way to obtain an advanced degree.

◆ *Study Helps*

1. Describe nursing as it existed in ancient civilizations.
2. Who was called the Father of Medicine, and why was he given this title?
3. How did the development of a middle class affect society and nursing in the Middle Ages?
4. Describe nursing during the Renaissance.
5. What contribution did St. Vincent de Paul make to the nursing profession?
6. Give a brief account of the life and activities of Florence Nightingale as they affected nursing.
7. What is the function of the Red Cross in the United States and abroad?
8. What were the chief contributions to nursing made by the following:
   - Dorothea Dix
   - Jean Dunant
   - Linda Richards
   - Clara Barton
   - Lillian Wald
   - Annie Goodrich
   - Mary Adelaid Nutting
   - Isabel Maitland Stewart
   - Isabel Hampton Robb
   - Hilda M. Torrop
   - Katherine Shepard
   - Etta Creech
   - Lillian Kuster
9. Which needs brought about the development of practical nursing?

Bibliography

Chaska NL: *The nursing profession: turning points,* St Louis, 1990, Mosby.
Dolan JA: *Nursing in society,* ed 15, Philadelphia, 1982, WB Saunders.
Donahue MP: *Nursing: the finest art,* St Louis, 1985, Mosby.
Fromer MJ: *Ethical issues in health care,* St Louis, 1981, Mosby.
Marriner-Tomey A: *Nursing theorists and their work,* St Louis, ed 2, 1989, Mosby.
Safier G: *Contemporary American leaders in nursing: an oral history,* New York, 1977, McGraw-Hill.
Saxton DF, Nugent PM, Pelikan PK: *Mosby's comprehensive review of nursing,* ed 13, St Louis, 1990, Mosby.

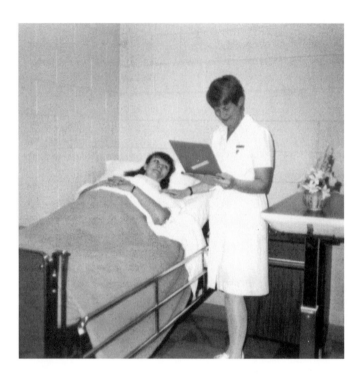

Objectives

At the completion of this chapter the student practical nurse will be able to:

◆ Discuss the classification system of hospitals.

◆ Identify members of the nursing team and discuss their roles.

◆ Elaborate on at least five nursing models.

◆ List and define the components of the nursing process.

4 Health Care Facilities and the Patient Care Team

◆ Hospitals

Purpose

Hospitals today have multiple functions. Most people's first thought of a hospital is as an institution designed to meet the needs of the sick and injured. But in the modern hospital there has been an expansion of medical knowledge, technical equipment, and research. The modern hospital provides facilities for the education of physicians, nurses, technicians, social workers, dietitians, therapists, and other health care personnel. It has clinical and research laboratories and takes part in the prevention of disease and the promotion of health through outpatient clinics in the hospital and in the outlying community.

The number of hospitals has steadily grown, and they are now a big business, ranking third in the nation's top 10 industries. Approximately 5 million workers, including more than 1.5 million nurses, are employed in hospitals.

Classification

A hospital is classified according to ownership, type of service rendered, length of patient stay, and size.

Ownership may be governmental or private. Government hospitals are operated and owned by federal, state, county, or city divisions. Such hospitals include those operated by the Veterans Administration, the Bureau of Indian Affairs, and the U.S. Public Health Service.

Privately owned hospitals are those owned and operated by labor unions, churches, business or industrial corporations, partners, or individuals. Many hospitals are non-profit organizations. Hospitals established to ensure profit are called *proprietary* hospitals.

Governmental and private institutions are further classified by service, for example, psychiatric, geriatric, general, and other special fields of medicine. They are sub-classified according to the number of beds available: fewer than 25 beds, 25 to 49, 50 to

99, 100 to 199, 200 to 299, 300 to 399, 400 to 499, and 500 beds or more. Federal-operated and state-operated hospitals frequently have the highest bed capacities, totaling 500 or more beds. The largest number of nonprofit hospitals fall into the 100- to 199-bed category; city and county hospitals are usually in the 50- to 99-bed category.

When hospitals are classified according to length of stay, they are divided into short term (less than 30 days), long term (30 days or longer), or a combination of both. Short-term institutions far outnumber long-term institutions. Hospitals are using community health facilities to decrease the number of hospital days and the financial cost to patients, institutions, and taxpayers.

As a result of increasing demands for hospital enlargement and remodeling, federal funds are available to individual hospitals under certain conditions. The Civil Rights Act, passed January 3, 1965, assures citizens that hospitals receiving federal funds are not operated on a segregated or discriminatory basis with regard to race, creed, color, or national origin. It is the primary function of the U.S. Public Health Service to ensure hospital compliance with signed statements of operation.

The National Health Planning and Resources Development Act of 1974 served as the legal basis for a not-for-profit corporation to be designated and funded by the U.S. Department of Health, Education, and Welfare (U.S. Department of Health and Human Services) as the official health planning and resource development agency for an area. The primary objective of the agency is to provide effective health planning for residents of the health service area. Effective health planning is an activity that identifies health needs and proposes ways to improve the availability, accessibility, and quality of care while being careful to control rising health care costs.

Diagnosis Related Groups

Diagnosis related groups (DRGs) are the result of the federal government's attempt to curb health costs. In the past the federal government reimbursed hospitals for a certain percentage of the cost incurred for caring for Medicare patients. This reimbursement continued for as long as the patients were hospitalized. Now, with the DRG system, the government specifies in advance how much of the hospital bill it will pay for these patients. The amount paid depends on the initial diagnosis, made when the patient is admitted to the hospital. Age, surgery, and complications are considered and can change the allotted period of confinement.

Major diagnostic categories have been established. Each category consists of specific diagnoses, and each diagnosis is assigned a DRG code number. The government has determined the length of hospital stay for a patient in that category. If a hospital discharges a patient before the allotted time, it keeps the profit made from the actual cost of caring for the patient and the amount paid by the government. If the patient stays longer than the allotted time, the hospital suffers a loss. DRGs are expected to save the government millions of dollars in Medicare payments.

Because of continuing changes, such as the DRG system, nurses need to develop more skills in business and management. Fewer personnel and more acutely ill patients necessitate utilization of available personnel to their fullest potential. Maintaining a close relationship with the medical records department and maintaining contact with physicians to assure records are complete and accurate become important and necessary functions for the nurse.

Administration

The ultimate governing body of any hospital is known as the *board of directors* or *trustees*. This board defines the philosophy of the institution (for example, to ensure patient care at the lowest possible cost) and its roles and functions, which include patient care, education, research, and community involvement.

The board delegates the administration of the hospital to an administrator or executive director. The administrator or director is responsible for managing the affairs of the hospital, business, and health care. The administrator may or may not have an assistant. In many hospitals an administrative council and medical director function in an assisting or advisory capacity to the administrator or director. The administrative council is composed of designated persons who collectively have the responsibility for all areas in the hospital, nursing and nonnursing. The medical director is responsible for the supervision and practice of the medical staff, interns, and residents. These functions may vary among different institutions.

Department heads govern major areas of operation. Each department head has assistants or supervisors who are responsible for the activities of several areas within a department. A key person is appointed in each specific area to assist the supervisor in carrying out the functions of the department. In the nursing areas this person is called the *head nurse*. The head nurse is directly responsible for patients, nursing care, and personnel in a particular division of the hospital. The head nurse appoints *team leaders,* who assign, guide, and assist team members in the performance of nursing procedures and treatments for the patient. Each has the responsibility for the activities of team members. Team members consist of registered and practical nurses, students, and ancillary personnel. Student practical nurses working as team members render patient care. Their assignments, guidance, and supervision, however, are the responsibility of the practical nurse instructor.

Educational Programs

Educational programs established for medical students, interns, and residents are under the direction of the medical director. In-service educational programs are under the direction of an in-service or educational coordinator. The director of the school of nursing is responsible for the faculty, students, and school curriculum. The faculty consists of instructors, clinical instructors, or a combination of both. The instructor usually teaches basic principles. The clinical instructor implements the application of principles in clinical practice in specific nursing areas. In programs that combine the two, one person functions as instructor and clinical instructor.

The in-service coordinator or educational director may be responsible to the director of nursing or to one of the administrative council members. The director of the school of nursing is frequently responsible to a member of the administrative council.

Accreditation

Hospital accreditation protects patients and grants recognition to hospitals for services rendered. It stimulates and urges hospitals to conduct ongoing self-evaluation within its structures to initiate continual growth and improvement. Accreditation requires institutions to meet specific standards that include good medical records, quality nursing care, organized medical staff, and adequate clinical facilities.

The accreditation committee consists of representatives from the American College of Physicians, American College of Surgeons, American Medical Association, and American Hospital Association. Surveys are conducted by field representatives, who report their findings to hospital representatives with suggestions for improvement at the termination of the survey and submit a detailed written report to the Board of Commissioners of the Joint Commission on Accreditation of Hospitals. Accreditation provides a means of improving hospital structure, organization, care, and employee morale and of ensuring quality care to patients.

◆ Nursing Team

Hospitals, extended care facilities, welfare agencies, and general health facilities have undergone great changes in education, function, and use of nursing personnel. These changes were necessary to keep pace with new demands in the health field. These new demands include medical and scientific advances, shorter hospital stays, and more complex nursing procedures. Although the supply of nurses is increasing to meet these demands, a shortage of personnel still exists in some areas.

The members of the nursing team included under nursing service today are registered and practical nurses, student nurses, nursing assistants, unit or ward clerks, and in some hospitals, ward or unit managers. Each of these hospital personnel gives either direct or indirect patient care. Indirect nursing care is performed away from the patient; direct nursing care is performed at the bedside. Through improved educational programs and in-service educational programs, the supply of better-prepared nursing personnel is constantly increasing.

Registered Nurse

It is important to know the role of the registered nurse to understand more completely your role as a practical nurse. There are similarities and differences between the two roles.

The registered nurse is a graduate of a college or university nursing program. The program may vary from 18 months to 4 years. The registered nurse has met the legal requirements for registration in the state of practice. This includes successful completion of a written examination, which demonstrates that the nurse possesses necessary technical knowledge and skill. Registered nurses may serve in various positions such as director of nursing service, supervisor, clinician, nurse practitioner, head nurse, staff nurse, or team leader, or they may be employed in private duty, physicians' offices, public health, or industry. Statistics show that the largest number of registered nurses are employed in hospitals.

The registered nurse assumes the responsibility for patient care in the absence of the physician. This responsibility has been entrusted by the hospital or institution, the attending physician, or both. The nurse's duty is to know the physical, spiritual, psychologic, and social status of each patient. Each nurse is expected to observe and report, as necessary, any significant symptoms or reactions in a patient and must see that all prescribed treatments and medications ordered by the physician are given.

As a staff nurse or team leader the registered nurse is directly responsible to the head nurse or, if entrusted with a higher position, the next person in the line of authority. The staff nurse or team leader must teach and supervise fellow team members, make assignments, and coordinate the activities of all personnel in that unit. The patient must be provided quality nursing care through a well-organized, smoothly functioning relationship among team members.

Practical Nurse

After you finish your program of practical nursing, you are eligible to take the licensing examination in the state where you are studying or in any state or U.S. territory, if you meet the established criteria of that state or territory. Success in passing this examination gives you the title of licensed practical nurse (LPN). This title means that you are a qualified practitioner of nursing, having completed the requirements in an approved program of practical nursing.

A few of the older licensed practical nurses received their licensure by waiver, meaning that they successfully passed the licensure examination even though they did not attend or complete an accredited program in practical nursing. Their past experiences in the field of practical nursing gave them sufficient knowledge to pass the licensure examination. This situation is nonexistent in all states today. Because of the high educational standards currently existing and because of the availability of approved schools of practical nursing, licensure is granted only after the applicant has completed an approved program in practical nursing and has successfully written the state board examination. Because nursing is a scientific and skilled profession, it demands qualified practitioners of nursing to ensure that the patient and his family receive safe and efficient nursing care.

Although programs vary somewhat in different states, the fundamental principles of practical nursing are included in all programs. Plans and ideas are being considered today to establish more uniformity in practical nursing requirements and to establish a universal recognition and acceptance of practical nurses.

You will in all probability be given tasks or functions to perform that require considerable skill and responsibility. An example may be the administration of medications. Remember that certain medications are administered by the licensed practical nurse, but other drugs, more potent and dangerous, are not. Licensed practical nurses are responsible for all their actions. If you assume a position for which you have not been trained, you are liable for your actions. Your particular state legislates laws concerning the functions you may perform as a licensed practical nurse. If you violate these laws, your license may be revoked by the state, and you may be prosecuted.

Statistics show that a majority of recently graduated practical nurses are employed by nursing homes, extended care facilities, home health agencies, and hospitals. By utilizing all members of the health care team to their maximum capacity, these facilities ensure safe, efficient, and effective nursing care for the public.

Student Nurse

The student nurse may be enrolled in either a registered nursing program or a practical nursing program. Both types of programs must provide good teaching situations. The student of a registered nursing program should be entrusted with responsible positions on the team for both learning and teaching experiences. However, she must be capable of handling this type of situation before it is given to her. She may function first as a team member and then as a team leader in clinical settings. In this type of learning experience the registered nurse is often assigned as a team member. In this position the registered nurse is readily available to assist the student in any difficult situations that arise. It gives the student nurse the assurance needed in this new experience, and it safeguards the patient's right to safe, quality nursing care.

As a practical nursing student you should be given situations that require direct nursing care of the patient and include various types of procedures. As a student working under the supervision of the registered nurse or licensed physician, you must learn which observations to make, their significance, and the importance of reporting them to the registered nurse, team leader, or physician. Because you work directly with the patient, you are in a position to observe the patient more closely and to discover his feelings about and reactions to his illness and treatment. With your assistance the registered nurse is more effective, since each team member is depended on to provide information. Your help is needed in caring for the patient. You need adequate supervision to receive instructions, interpret orders, and learn to perform procedures correctly. In this manner you can give competent bedside care without causing harm or distress to either your patient or yourself.

Nursing Assistant

The nursing assistant is assigned to provide simple nursing care and to perform uncomplicated nursing procedures. She is assigned to either male or female patients.

The nursing assistant gives direct care to less seriously ill patients and assists practical nurses and registered nurses in rendering care to critically ill patients. She is prepared for her position through in-service classes and on-the-job training. Some hospitals have a 2- to 6-week nursing assistant program. Each assistant must attend this program and successfully pass an examination before being permitted to work in the clinical area as a team member.

These employees are taught fundamental principles and procedures such as bedmaking; bathing a patient; ambulation; afternoon and evening care; taking blood pressure, temperature, pulse, and respiration; and the method of distributing fresh drinking water. Formerly, many cleaning duties such as washing beds and units after the patient's discharge and cleaning closets and utility rooms were assigned to the nursing assistant. Today in most hospitals the housekeeping department has taken over these duties. This frees the nursing assistant to spend more time with the patient and to render additional nursing care.

Unit or Ward Clerk

The unit or ward clerk is usually considered one of the clerical nursing personnel. This employee has clerical, administrative, hostess, and public relations duties to perform, as well as much of the paper and desk work. The unit or ward clerk keeps the nursing station area in good order and appearance and coordinates communications for the registered nurse and team members. The unit clerk is prepared to free the nurse from time-consuming paper work by ordering supplies, making out necessary requisitions, processing physicians' orders, and taking and answering telephone messages other than those involving physicians' orders.

It is helpful if the unit clerk has some secretarial experience and on-the-job training to be more organized and systematic in fulfilling the duties of the job of unit clerk. The unit or ward clerk is frequently responsible to the head nurse. However, if a unit manager is used in the hospital, the ward clerk may be responsible to the unit manager.

Unit Manager

The position of unit manager is being used in some hospitals; the responsibilities are administrative and are planned to free the nursing personnel for patient care.

The unit manager contacts other hospital departments such as the housekeeping, pharmacy, and dietary departments; is responsible for most of the nonnursing duties on the unit; and answers to the unit coordinator, who is directly accountable to the administrator or administrative assistant.

◆ Nursing Care Models

The interest of every hospital is to render quality, efficient, and economical nursing care. The nursing care model depends on the hospital and the use of the personnel previously discussed. Nursing care models are created as a result of patients' needs, and they should be given much consideration. There are three general methods of assignment: the functional patient care method, the comprehensive patient care method, and the progressive patient care method.

Functional Patient Care

The functional patient care method is one in which personnel are assigned specific duties such as giving baths, performing treatments, dispensing medications, and starting intravenous fluids. This is the oldest acceptable method of giving nursing care; however, it is not necessarily the best method. With this method the registered nurse has certain duties such as checking physicians' orders; the practical nurse gives treatments; and the nursing assistant gives baths and makes beds. Only a cross section of ward activities is seen in this type of assignment method, and patient care is sporadic and often unorganized.

Comprehensive, Primary Care, and Team Nursing

Comprehensive nursing. In the comprehensive method the nurse has the complete care of all patients assigned for a given shift. This method includes actual bedside care, spiritual and mental needs, and teaching the patient to cope with his condition in the hospital and when he goes home. With this method the nurse has an opportunity to know the patient as completely as possible. Therefore in comprehensive patient care the patient is considered a complete individual, and all aspects of his care are administered by the same nurse.

Primary care nursing. Primary care nursing is similar to comprehensive nursing in that one nurse is assigned to each patient. The difference between the two is in the length of time the nurse is responsible for the patient's care.

The primary care nurse is a registered nurse and is the principal nurse for the patient. She is responsible for planning the 24-hour nursing care of several patients from the day they are admitted to the hospital to the day they are discharged. The primary care nurse assesses the needs of the patient and together with the patient and other health care personnel formulates a nursing care plan. The primary nurse should be able to demonstrate advanced knowledge and skill. These are generally attained through work experience and continuing education. The primary nurse must have authority, accountability, and autonomy in patient care, and her clinical nursing practice should set an example for other members of the health team.

The associate nurse may be a registered nurse or a licensed practical nurse who has been approved by the head nurse and who has the knowledge and skill to provide direct and total patient care. The associate nurse must be able to follow a nursing care plan, identify the changes that may occur in a patient's condition to alter the planned interventions, and correctly document patient responses. The associate nurse serves as the right hand of the primary care nurse, and together they work to provide total holistic care to the patients on their unit.

Team nursing. The team method of assignment is probably the most widely used method today. It provides for the maximum use of all employees' abilities for an assigned group of patients. Team members have total responsibility for these patients. The team may be under the direction of a registered nurse, a licensed practical nurse, or a student nurse from a registered nursing program. The team consists of the team leader, or director, and team members. These members include a registered nurse or nurses, licensed practical nurses, student nurses, and nursing assistants.

The purpose of team nursing is to render quality nursing care to a specified group of patients by using each member of the team to the fullest capacity. The team leader is familiar with all the patients assigned to the team and their disease processes, knows the team members and their capabilities, and plans assignments with this knowledge in mind. The team leader may incorporate both the functional and comprehensive methods of nursing care.

Depending on the type of personnel and their training, the team leader may use the comprehensive method, assigning each team member the total care of particular patients. This service includes medications, treatments, and nursing care. This method may not be advisable to use when the team consists of nursing assistants because they do not have the proper training to perform some of these functions.

The functional method, in a modified form, is often the most commonly used method. The team leader or one of the registered nurses is assigned to administer the medications to all patients assigned to the team. Treatment and nursing care are given by individual team members for all assigned patients. The team leader or registered nurse may be required to perform advanced or difficult procedures or at least supervise or assist in their performance.

A description of the daily routine of a hospital shift (7 AM to 3:30 PM) using the team method may be as follows:

The team leader receives the report on all patients from the night nurse at 7 AM.

The team leader then adjusts the assignments for personnel. It is advisable to make these assignments the evening or day before.

The team leader checks all patients briefly.

While the leader is performing these activities, the team members are preparing patients for breakfast and serving them their trays.

At 8 AM the team leader gives assignments to team members, including reports on all patients assigned to them.

Team members render the designated nursing care and perform treatments as ordered. They seek assistance if and when necessary.

The team leader administers medications and assists with treatments as necessary.

The team members give feedback of any pertinent information to the team leader.

After morning care has been completed and lunch trays have been served, the leader has a conference with the team members. The conference may be centered around one patient, or it may be a brief report on all or selected patients. It should indicate the patient's needs and possible suggestions made by the group for planning the care of the patient, which are recorded on the written nursing care plans.

This conference is necessary. It helps the team members to realize their importance on the team. It stimulates their interest and encourages them to give better care. It gives them a clearer understanding of their patient as a total individual. It helps the team leader to plan the patient's care. It assists the team leader in knowing the patient and his needs more thoroughly and in discovering significant factors relating to his treatment and care. It helps to gain the understanding, confidence, and support of all team members.

After treatments have been completed, the patients made comfortable, and rooms put in proper order, members make a final check on the medical record to ensure that nothing has been forgotten or omitted.

At 3 PM the team leader gives a report on all patients to the oncoming registered nurse.

The team method requires the total effort and active participation of all its members.

Progressive Patient Care

Progressive patient care is a concept in which medical and nursing care is carried out according to the degree of illness and the patient's needs, instead of according to cost, sex, and diagnosis. Depending on the hospital, these needs are broken down into five units, or divisions. Each unit is designed to meet the needs of the individual patient.

Intensive care unit. The intensive care unit is designed to care for critically ill patients. Their conditions may be the result of injuries, surgery, or disease. These patients receive specialized nursing care by trained staff. Often in this area the team method of assignment is used. These units have necessary drugs and lifesaving equipment readily available. A nurse with maturity, good health, emotional stability, and ability to work well under pressure is an asset to this division. A patient is transferred from the intensive care area by written or verbal orders of the attending physician when he believes that the patient no longer requires this type of nursing care.

Intermediate care unit. The intermediate care unit is designed for patients who need a moderate amount of nursing care. Some of these patients are able to help plan and carry out part of their care, such as taking their own baths, being up and about or at least walking to the bathroom, and taking care of their own personal needs.

The procedures performed by health care personnel are of a more routine nature. The functional assignment method may be effective in this area. However, many hospitals today are using the team method.

Teaching in this area is of utmost importance to prepare the patient adequately for the self-care unit. The emotional and physical reactions to illness must be understood by the nurse on this unit to prepare the patient for the future.

Combination of intensive care and intermediate care units. Some hospitals are now combining the two types of care to ensure a continuity of medical care and to provide a complete learning situation for the medical personnel receiving training.

Same day surgery unit. Patients admitted to the same day surgery (SDS) unit are those who have surgical procedures performed in which the anesthesia department may be involved, either general, intravenous, regional, or monitored anesthesia care.

Patients are admitted in the morning, 2 hours before the scheduled surgery. The patient may have blood work done that morning or may have had blood work done during the previous week. The SDS patient has surgery and goes home by 6 PM or after recovery. If there is a complication, the patient is admitted to an observation unit and may remain in the hospital for 23 hours. Observation and SDS patients are considered outpatients.

Nurses working in these units must have the following:
1. Skills in pre- and postoperative assessment of the surgical patient.
2. Skills in the use of emergency equipment and procedures.
3. Teaching skills enabling them to provide pre- and postoperative instructions to the patient and the family.

Day of surgery admission. Day of surgery admission (DOSA) is for patients who are admitted on the morning of surgery, have major surgery, and stay in the hospital for several days or as long as needed. Hysterectomy and cholecystectomy are examples of surgeries for which this procedure is used.

Long-term care unit. The long-term care unit may also be known as the extended care unit. The patients in this unit require nursing care over an extended period of time. The functional or team method of nursing care may be used in this area.

The care of these patients may require the use of more nonprofessional personnel, supervised by the registered nurse, rather than professional help. Teaching and rehabilitation are important for the patient's satisfactory return home. Recreational and occupational therapy are stressed in this unit.

Other Types of Nursing Care

Community health nursing. Community health centers are established in an effort to bring health care into the communities. They are designed to motivate the poor and deprived to seek care freely. The community health nurse provides many types of patient care in such centers.

Some types of health care provided are (1) prenatal care for maternity patients; (2) psychiatric care such as day care, therapy groups, foster family care, halfway houses, and night care centers; and (3) rehabilitative care, which serves mostly young persons, many of whom are treated for drug addiction. There are also centers for vagrants, where many middle-aged and older persons receive necessary care.

Although the scope and boundaries of these community services vary and still remain issues for continued exploration and improvement, with this type of health care available in the neighborhoods more people have access to and receive the care they need.

Home health care agencies. The purpose of home health care agencies is to provide home care services essential for maintaining persons at home in the presence of illness or disability. Services are directed toward preservation and restoration of health, prevention of disease and disability, and therapeutic care and rehabilitation on an intermittent basis in an individual's place of residence. Services are rendered by licensed registered nurses, licensed practical nurses, social workers, dietitians, home health aides, physical therapists, occupational therapists, speech therapists, and other appropriate personnel.

Hospice unit and care. Hospices arose as a reaction to the tried way of caring for the terminally ill patient. The hospice idea tries to overcome the inhumane approach by portraying death and dying as inevitable and normal. To be admitted to a hospice usually requires that a patient have 6 months or less to live. Control over the patient's illness, care, and environment are maintained. Within the hospice unit, patients and their families are looked on as one complete unit requiring care. Nurses are able to establish a close relationship with the patient and the family. This allays many of the patient's fears, assists him to die with dignity, and comforts the family members in their time of bereavement.

Private duty nursing. The private duty nurse takes care of each patient on an individual basis. This care may be in an institution, a home, or wherever the patient desires. It may include traveling with the patient. The nurse is paid by the patient or the family and is directly responsible to the patient's physician. If the patient is in an institution, the nurse is responsible also to the nursing administration.

◆ Tools of Nursing Care

Quality nursing care is the goal of every hospital. Its achievement requires using personnel to their fullest potential and planning and evaluating nursing care.

The admission nursing assessment/history form (Fig. 4–1), discharge orders/summary form (Fig. 4–2), and short stay nursing admission form (Fig. 4–3) are three useful tools, when used correctly, to assist you in meeting your patient's needs.

The nursing care plan is a decision-making process. It is a problem-solving technique and when applied to a nursing situation is frequently referred to as the *nursing*

**ADMISSION NURSING
ASSESSMENT/
HISTORY**

PATIENT LABEL

ALLERGY/SENSITIVITY: (FOOD/DRUG)   SYMPTOMS:

ALLERGIES: ❑ STICKER ON CHART ❑ RECORDED ON MED SHEET
❑ PHARMACY NOTIFIED ❑ DIETARY NOTIFIED ❑ I.D. BAND ON

DATE _____ TIME _____

PATIENT _____ INFORMANT _____

*AGE _____ *RACE _____ T _____ P _____ R _____ BP _____ HEIGHT _____ WEIGHT_____

ADMISSION DIAGNOSIS _____

CHIEF COMPLAINT _____

DR. _____ NOTIFIED.   DATE _____ TIME _____

PAST MEDICAL HISTORY (Example: diabetes, heart disease, hepatitis, anemia, hypertension, etc.)

MEDICAL _____   SURGICAL _____

_____   _____

_____   _____

TRAUMATIC INJURIES _____   _____

_____   **(*If cancer, year diagnosed/site)** _____

PRESENT MEDICATIONS (Dosage and time)

_____   _____

_____   _____

_____   _____

DO YOU USE MOOD ALTERING CHEMICALS? ❑ YES ❑ NO IF YES, LIST _____

MEDICATIONS: ❑ HOME ❑ BEDSIDE ❑ SECURITY   _____

*ALCOHOL (Duration/Amount/Day) _____   *SMOKING (Duration/Amount/Day) _____

    1. HAVE YOU EVER FELT YOU SHOULD CUT DOWN ON YOUR DRINKING? ❑ YES ❑ NO

    2. HAVE PEOPLE ANNOYED YOU BY CRITICIZING YOUR DRINKING? ❑ YES ❑ NO

    3. HAVE YOU EVER FELT BAD OR GUILTY ABOUT YOUR DRINKING? ❑ YES ❑ NO

    4. HAVE YOU EVER HAD A DRINK FIRST THING WHEN YOU AWAKENED TO STEADY YOUR NERVES OR
       TO GET RID OF A HANGOVER? ❑ YES ❑ NO

FAMILY MEDICAL HISTORY (Include grandparents, parents, siblings)

DIABETES _____   **CANCER** (Site) _____

TUBERCULOSIS _____   HYPERTENSION _____

HEART DISEASE _____   ANEMIA _____

SIGNATURE _____

Fig. 4-1   Courtesy St Mary's Health Center, St Louis, Missouri.

NEURO/CEREBRAL FUNCTION

Alterations in thought processes.
Alterations in communications.
Potential for violence.

❑ **WNL** ❑ DECREASED ATTENTION SPAN ❑ ALTERED PERCEPTION ❑ TREMORS

❑ FAMILY REPORTS CHANGE IN BEHAVIOR ❑ IMPAIRED MEMORY ❑ SEIZURES

❑ IMPAIRED JUDGEMENT ❑ PARESTHESIAS ❑ ATAXIA ❑ CONFUSION ❑ COMATOSE

❑ COMBATIVE ❑ RESTLESSNESS ❑ PARALYSIS ❑ HEADACHES ❑ SPEECH DIFFICULTY

COMMENTS _____

COGNITIVE RESPONSE

Lack of knowledge.

INEXPERIENCE WITH: ❑ THERAPY ❑ DISEASE ❑ HOSPITALIZATION

BARRIERS TO LEARNING: ❑ LANGUAGE ❑ VISION ❑ HEARING ❑ LITERACY

❑ OTHER ❑ ASKS QUESTIONS/REQUESTS INFORMATION

TEACHING AIDS REQUIRED _____

COMMENTS _____

COMFORT

Alterations in comfort.
Alterations in sleeping pattern.

❑ **WNL** ❑ PAIN _____

EXACERBATED BY _____

RELIEVED BY _____

❑ SLEEP DISTURBANCES/SLEEPING AIDS _____

COMMENTS _____

RESPIRATORY

Ineffective airway clearance.
Ineffective breathing patterns.
Impaired gas exchange.

❑ **WNL** ❑ DYSPNEA ❑ COUGH ❑ SPUTUM ❑ PLEURITIC PAIN ❑ HOARSENESS

❑ USES HOME O_2 _____ L/MIN

LUNG SOUNDS _____

COMMENTS _____

CIRCULATORY

Decreased cardiac output.
Alteration in peripheral tissue perfusion.
Alterations in fluid volume.

❑ **WNL** ❑ VERTIGO ❑ PALPITATIONS ❑ SYNCOPE ❑ KNOWN MURMUR ❑ CHEST PAIN

❑ HYPERTENSION ❑ LEG CRAMPS ❑ VARICOSITIES ❑ EDEMA

COMMENTS _____

IMMUNE FUNCTION

Potential for infection.
Alteration in body temperature.

❑ **WNL** ❑ CHRONIC DISEASE ❑ TRANSPLANT ❑ RADIATION ❑ STEROIDS

❑ CHEMOTHERAPY ❑ INVASIVE DEVICE/INTERNAL PROSTHESIS ❑ CHILLS

❑ INCREASED TEMP ❑ DECREASED TEMP

COMMENTS _____

NUTRITION

Alterations in nutrition.

❑ **WNL** DIET _____

❑ DECREASED APPETITE ❑ INCREASED APPETITE ❑ DIFFICULTY CHEWING

❑ DYSPHAGIA ❑ NAUSEA/VOMITING ❑ RECENT WEIGHT LOSS/GAIN _____ LBS.

COMMENTS _____

GASTROINTESTINAL

Alterations in bowel elimination.

❑ **WNL** DATE OF LAST BM _____ ❑ CONSTIPATION ❑ DIARRHEA

❑ HEMORRHOIDS ❑ FLATULENCE ❑ ABDOMINAL PAIN ❑ CRAMPS ❑ OSTOMY

BOWEL SOUNDS _____

COMMENTS _____

URINARY

Alterations in urinary elimination.

❑ **WNL** ❑ FREQUENCY ❑ URGENCY ❑ INCONTINENCE ❑ POLYURIA ❑ DYSURIA

❑ HEMATURIA ❑ NOCTURIA ❑ CALCULI ❑ RETENTION ❑ CATHETER ❑ OSTOMY

COMMENTS _____

Continued

REPRODUCTIVE SEXUALITY

Alterations in sexual function/response.

FEMALE: *MENSTRUAL HISTORY: AGE OF ONSET _____ LMP _____
DATE OF LAST PAP SMEAR _____ ❏ VAGINAL DISCHARGE ❏ STD ❏ PID
*PREGNANCIES _____ *LIVE BIRTHS _____
POST-MENOPAUSAL: MENOPAUSE AGE _____ ❏ BLEEDING
BREAST: ❏ MASSES ❏ TENDERNESS ❏ DISCHARGE
DATE OF LAST MAMMOGRAMS: _____
MALE: ❏ WNL ❏ PENILE DISCHARGE ❏ LESIONS ❏ STD ❏ PROSTATE ENLARGEMENT
TESTICLES: ❏ MASSES ❏ PAIN ❏ SWELLING
COMMENTS _____

MUSCULOSKELETAL

Impaired physical mobility.
Self-care deficit.
Activity intolerance.

❏ WNL ❏ FATIGUE ❏ DECREASED STRENGTH ❏ IMPAIRED COORDINATION ❏ PAIN
❏ SWELLING ❏ DEFORMITY ❏ FALL HISTORY ❏ ABNORMAL GAIT ❏ LIMITED MOTION
❏ WEIGHT BEARING LIMITATIONS ❏ STIFFNESS ❏ LIMITATIONS/DISABILITIES
❏ ASSISTIVE DEVICES _____
COMMENTS _____

SKIN/MUCOUS MEMBRANES

Impaired skin integrity.
Alterations in oral mucous membranes.

❏ WNL COLOR/TEMP _____ ❏ REDNESS ❏ DIAPHORESIS ❏ ITCHING ❏ WOUND ❏ BREAKDOWN
❏ LESIONS/RASH ❏ POOR TURGOR ❏ ECCHYMOSIS ❏ BODY SECRETIONS/ODOR ❏ SORE THROAT
DESCRIPTION _____
CONDITION OF MOUTH _____
DISCHARGE FROM: ❏ EYES ❏ EARS ❏ NOSE
COMMENTS _____

PT. STATUS	ASSESSMENT OF DECUBITUS ULCER POTENTIAL							SCORE
GENERAL STATE OF HEALTH	GOOD	0	FAIR	1	POOR	2	VERY BAD	3	
MENTAL STATUS	ALERT	0	LETHARGIC	1	SEMI-COMATOSE	2	COMATOSE	3	
ACTIVITY	AMBULATORY	0	NEED HELP	1	CHAIRFAST	4	BEDFAST	6	
MOBILITY	FULL	0	LIMITED	1	VERY LIMITED	4	IMMOBILE	6	
INCONTINENCE	NONE	0	OCCASIONAL	1	USUALLY URINE	4	URINE/FECES	6	
ORAL NUTRI-TIONAL INTAKE	GOOD	0	FAIR	1	POOR	2	NONE	3	

0 - 4 = NOT AT RISK	12 OR GREATER = INITIATE DECUBITUS PREVENTION PROGRAM	❏ MULTIPLE OR DEEP DECUBITUS PRESENT = INITIATE DECUBITUS FLOW SHEET	
5 - 11 = MODERATE RISK Reassess in 5 days	Reassess q̄ 7 days		TOTAL ► SCORE _____

EMOTIONAL RESPONSE

Alterations in coping.
Alterations in self-control.
Anxiety/fear.
Dysfunctional grieving.

VERBALIZES: ❏ **NO CONCERNS VERBALIZED** ❏ LOW MOOD ❏ FEAR ❏ CHRONIC WORRY
❏ LOSS OF CONTROL ❏ INABILITY TO COPE/PROBLEM SOLVE ❏ ANXIOUS ❏ ANGRY
❏ APPREHENSIVE ❏ CRYING ❏ IRRITABLE ❏ SELF-NEGLECT
❏ LACK OF EYE CONTACT ❏ WITHDRAWN
❏ LOSS OR CHANGE IN STRUCTURE/FUNCTION OF BODY PART ❏ RECENT LOSS
COMMENTS _____

SAFETY

Potential for injury.

❏ VISION PROBLEMS ❏ GLASSES ❏ CONTACTS ❏ PROSTHESIS ❏ GLAUCOMA
❏ CATARACTS ❏ HEARING PROBLEMS ❏ HEARING AID ❏ FALL ALERT BAND APPLIED
COMMENTS _____
RISK FACTORS FOR INJURY _____
PATIENT INSTRUCTED: ❏ NURSE'S CALL LIGHT/EMERGENCY/TV/PHONE/BED ❏ SMOKING POLICY

FALL RISK ASSESSMENT

PATIENT STATUS	0	1	2	POINTS
CLINICAL STATUS	HEALTHY (ADMITTED FOR ACUTE EPISODE)	POTENTIAL FOR MILD DEBILITATION (POST OP)	ILLNESS RELATED DEBILITATION	
MENTAL STATUS	ALERT AND ORIENTED X 3	APATHETIC WITH SHORT TERM MEMORY	FRANK CONFUSION OR HALLUCINATING	
CONTINENCE	FULLY CONTINENT	FOLEY CATHETER	FREQUENCY, DIARRHEA, INCONTINENCE	
MOBILITY	FULLY AMBULATORY	SLOW GAIT, HOLDS FURNITURE	UNSTEADY GAIT, NEEDS ASSIST TO WALK, MOBILITY AIDS	
AGE	65 AND UNDER	OVER 94	66 - 93	
MEDICATIONS	NO MEDS	ANY MEDS	CNS DEPRESSANTS, SEDATIVES, ANESTHESIA, ALCOHOL	
FALL HISTORY		NO FALL HISTORY	HISTORY OF FALLS	

0 - 4 = NO FALL RISK	5 OR GREATER = INITIATE FALL PREVENTION PROGRAM	TOTAL ► POINTS _____

VALUABLES			
☐ POLICY EXPLAINED	SECURITY	PATIENT	HOME
DENTURES			
RINGS			
WATCH			
MONEY			
PROSTHESIS			
GLASSES			
OTHER			

ORGAN DONATION
☐ YES   ☐ NO
☐ ANY ORGAN
☐ SPECIFIC ORGAN
_____

PERSON TO NOTIFY IN CASE OF EMERGENCY
NAME _____
RELATIONSHIP _____
TELEPHONE NUMBER _____

ADVANCE DIRECTIVES/LIVING WILL
HAS PATIENT/FAMILY RECEIVED BROCHURE?   ☐ YES   ☐ NO
DOES PATIENT HAVE ADVANCE DIRECTIVES/LIVING WILL?   ☐ YES   ☐ NO
COPY OF ADVANCE DIRECTIVE/LIVING WILL IN CHART?   ☐ YES   ☐ NO

SOCIAL SYSTEM/ DISCHARGE PLANNING

Alteration in family processes.
Social isolation.
Spiritual distress.

MARITAL STATUS: ☐ S ☐ M ☐ SEP ☐ D ☐ W   INSURANCE: ☐ YES ☐ NO

RELIGION _____ EDUCATIONAL BACKGROUND _____

*OCCUPATION _____ NUMBER OF YEARS _____

*IF RETIRED, PREVIOUS OCCUPATION _____

*EXPOSURE TO CARCINOGENS/TOXINS _____

LIVES: ☐ HOME ☐ ALONE ☐ WITH FAMILY ☐ ECF_____

SUPPORT PERSON _____ ☐ AVAILABLE FOR CARE AFTER DISCHARGE

FEELING OF: ☐ ALONENESS ☐ REJECTION ☐ BEING DIFFERENT FROM OTHERS

☐ OTHER _____

☐ FAMILY UNABLE TO MEET PHYSICAL/EMOTIONAL/SPIRITUAL NEEDS _____

HOME ENVIRONMENT AFFECTING CARE _____

COMMENTS _____

1) PREVIOUS COMMUNITY SERVICES PROVIDED (HOME HEALTH, MEALS ON WHEELS, INCLUDE NAME OF AGENCY OR SERVICE)
_____

2) POTENTIAL NEEDS/PROBLEMS IN THESE AREAS FOLLOWING DISCHARGE:

☐ TRANSPORTATION TO APP'T   ☐ MED INSTRUCTIONS   ☐ NEWLY DIAGNOSED/INSTRUCTIONS
☐ THERAPY (PT, OT, SPEECH, ETC.)   ☐ MOBILITY (STAIRS, ETC.)   ☐ DRESSING CHANGES
☐ HOMEMAKER CHORES   ☐ PERSONAL CARE   ☐ FINANCES
☐ EQUIPMENT NEEDS (O$_2$, PUMPS, BED, WALKER, ETC.)   ☐ OTHER _____

3) **REFERRALS MADE AT ADMISSION**

DEPT	DATE	NURSE REFERRING

SIGNATURE _____ DATE _____ TIME _____

CONTINUITY OF CARE CONFERENCES

DATES:								
DEPARTMENT PRESENT	☐ NURSING ☐ SOC SER ☐ HOME HEALTH ☐ PM&R ☐ DIETETICS	☐ UR ☐ SSMRI ☐ PAST.CARE ☐ NRSG.ED. ☐ SNU	☐ NURSING ☐ SOC SER ☐ HOME HEALTH ☐ PM&R ☐ DIETETICS	☐ UR ☐ SSMRI ☐ PAST.CARE ☐ NRSG.ED. ☐ SNU	☐ NURSING ☐ SOC SER ☐ HOME HEALTH ☐ PM&R ☐ DIETETICS	☐ UR ☐ SSMRI ☐ PAST.CARE ☐ NRSG.ED. ☐ SNU	☐ NURSING ☐ SOC SER ☐ HOME HEALTH ☐ PM&R ☐ DIETETICS	☐ UR ☐ SSMRI ☐ PAST.CARE ☐ NRSG.ED. ☐ SNU
CONFERENCE SUMMARY / REFERRALS MADE								

DISCHARGE ORDERS/SUMMARY

DATE: _____   DISCHARGE VITAL SIGNS: T _____ P _____ R _____ BP _____

DISCHARGE TO: ☐ Home ☐ Family ☐ Nursing Home _____

☐ Home Health ☐ Other Institution _____   ☐ Outpatient Therapy _____

DISCHARGE DIAGNOSIS: ☐ See DRG Sheet or face sheet. Primary _____

Secondary _____

	MEDICINE	DOSE	ROUTE	FREQUENCY
D				
I				
S				
C				
H				
A				
R				
G				
E				
M				
E				
D				
S				

TREATMENT INSTRUCTIONS: _____

_____

_____

_____

DIET: ☐ Regular ☐ Modified (specify) _____

ACTIVITY PERMITTED:
☐ No Restrictions
☐ Walking _____
☐ Driving _____
☐ Don't lift over _____ pounds
☐ Weight bearing _____

☐ Stairs _____
☐ Shower/Bath _____
☐ Work - Return in _____ days/weeks
☐ Other _____

FOLLOW-UP:
☐ Make an appointment to be seen in my office in _____ weeks, and Dr. _____ in _____ weeks.
☐ Appointment made to see Dr. _____ on _____ at _____ am / pm.
☐ Bring all medications to office.   ☐ Call office in _____

NURSING INSTRUCTIONS: _____

_____

Mode of Discharge _____   Valuables _____

PATIENT INSTRUCTIONS RECEIVED BY:

_____
M.D. SIGNATURE

_____
PATIENT OR RELATIONSHIP TO PATIENT

_____
R.N. SIGNATURE

F0820 (1/91)

Fig. 4-2   Courtesy St Mary's Health Center, St Louis, Missouri.

SHORT STAY
NURSING ADMISSION

PATIENT LABEL

ALLERGIES								

ADMISSION DATE		TIME		AGE			SEX ☐ M ☐ F	

T	P	R		B/P	HEIGHT	WEIGHT	

ADMISSION DIAGNOSIS

CHIEF COMPLAINT

M E D I C A L   H I S T O R Y   P A S T

MEDICAL	SURGICAL

TRAUMATIC INJURIES

CURRENT MEDICATIONS

HABITS ☐ SMOKING AMT/DAY _____ ☐ ALCOHOL AMT/DAY _____ DATE OF LAST BM

DIET

S Y S T E M I C   R E V I E W

NEURO/CEREBRAL
MENTAL STATUS
RESPIRATORY
CIRCULATORY
GASTROINTESTINAL
GENITOURINARY
MUSCULOSKELETAL

FALL RISK ASSESSMENT

PATIENT STATUS	0	1	2	POINTS
CLINICAL STATUS	HEALTHY (ADMITTED FOR ACUTE EPISODE)	POTENTIAL FOR MILD DEBILITATION (POST OP)	ILLNESS RELATED DEBILITATION	
MENTAL STATUS	ALERT AND ORIENTED X 3	APATHETIC WITH SHORT TERM MEMORY	FRANK CONFUSION OR HALLUCINATING	
CONTINENCE	FULLY CONTINENT	FOLEY CATHETER	FREQUENCY DIARRHEA, INCONTINENCE	
MOBILITY	FULLY AMBULATORY	SLOW GAIT, HOLDS FURNITURE	UNSTEADY GAIT, NEEDS ASSIST TO WALK, MOBILITY AIDS	
AGE	65 AND UNDER	OVER 94	66 - 93	
MEDICATIONS	NO MEDS	ANY MEDS	CNS DEPRESSANTS, SEDATIVES, ANESTHESIA, ALCOHOL	
FALL HISTORY		NO FALL HISTORY	HISTORY OF FALLS	

0 - 4 = NO FALL RISK	5 OR GREATER = INITIATE FALL PREVENTION PROGRAM	TOTAL ► POINTS _____

PT. STATUS	ASSESSMENT OF DECUBITUS ULCER POTENTIAL							SCORE
GENERAL STATE OF HEALTH	GOOD	0	FAIR	1	POOR	2	VERY BAD	3
MENTAL STATUS	ALERT	0	LETHARGIC	1	SEMI-COMATOSE	2	COMATOSE	3
ACTIVITY	AMBULATORY	0	NEED HELP	1	CHAIRFAST	4	BEDFAST	6
MOBILITY	FULL	0	LIMITED	1	VERY LIMITED	4	IMMOBILE	6
INCONTINENCE	NONE	0	OCCASIONAL	1	USUALLY URINE	4	URINE/FECES	6
ORAL NUTRI-TIONAL INTAKE	GOOD	0	FAIR	1	POOR	2	NONE	3

0 - 4 = NOT AT RISK 5 - 11 = MODERATE RISK Reassess in 5 days	12 OR GREATER = INITIATE DECUBITUS PREVENTION PROGRAM Reassess q 7 days	☐ MULTIPLE OR DEEP DECUBITUS PRESENT = INITIATE DECUBITUS FLOW SHEET	TOTAL ► SCORE _____

VALUABLES				
☐ POLICY EXPLAINED	SECURITY	PATIENT	HOME	
DENTURES				
RINGS				
WATCH				
MONEY				
PROSTHESIS				
GLASSES				
OTHER				

ORGAN DONATION

☐ YES   ☐ NO

☐ ANY ORGAN

☐ SPECIFIC ORGAN: _____

PERSON TO NOTIFY IN CASE OF EMERGENCY

NAME _____

RELATIONSHIP _____

TELEPHONE NO. _____

LIVING WILL / ADVANCE DIRECTIVES

HAS PATIENT/FAMILY RECEIVED BROCHURE? ☐ YES ☐ NO

DOES PATIENT HAVE ADVANCE DIRECTIVES/LIVING WILL? ☐ YES ☐ NO

COPY OF ADVANCE DIRECTIVE/LIVING WILL IN CHART? ☐ YES ☐ NO

SIGNATURE	DATE	TIME
REVIEWED BY RN	DATE	TIME
MD NOTIFIED	DATE	TIME

Fig. 4-3   Courtesy St Mary's Health Center, St Louis, Missouri.

process. The nursing process is the systematic, intelligent course of meeting patient problems. It describes the thoughts and behaviors of the nurses administering care to patients. It is a design for organizing nursing activity, a means to an end, and a process for understanding and promoting health.

The nursing process involves two people, the nurse and the patient. It is a dynamic communication process, and because of this process behaviors may be affected. For example, the behavior of the nurse may affect the patient, the behavior of the patient may affect the nurse, and the environment may affect both. The interaction process differs with each patient because each patient is an individual and with each nurse because of previous learning, experiences, values, and expectations.

The components of the nursing process are as follows:

1. *Assessment*—collecting information about the patient obtained from the nursing history, frequent patient observations, physical assessment, the nursing report, and the patient's medical record. With this knowledge base the nurse identifies problems the patient may be experiencing. Assessment is the continuous process by which nurses analyze what they feel, see, hear, and smell, and what the patient verbalizes. There are three general categories of patient problems:
   a. Actual problems that are observed and noted during the assessment
   b. Potential problems that the patient, because of the disease condition, has a high risk of developing
   c. Possible problems that require additional information before they are considered pertinent to the patient or ruled out as not relevant to the patient

2. *Planning*—developing the specific plan or method of care that involves realistic goal setting for the patient. Nursing approaches are planned to address the specific problems of the patient that have been identified according to priority of need. The nurse sets short-term goals for the patient's progress after determining the potential that exists for correcting the problems. The established level of recovery for the patient must be realistic. Short-term goals, or expected outcomes, are determined for each identified problem. Long-term goals are established in the form of discharge criteria or the progress of the patient in terms of the expected outcome of the disease and activities at the time of discharge.

3. *Implementation* (intervention)—initiating and carrying out of the plan that has been established. This means adhering to the plan according to the policies and procedures of the hospital in performing all nursing actions.

4. *Evaluation*—judging the effectiveness of the nursing approaches through examining the patient's responses to the care given. The plan must be revised if the desired effects are not being produced. Evaluation is a continuous process by which the nurse judges the effectiveness of each approach and adapts a plan of care to the patient's responses.

The components of the nursing process may at times be labeled differently, but they are always present. Regardless of labels, the nursing process promotes a systematized, organized way of thinking. The nursing process guides the nurse in decision making, communication, and problem solving. It is a means to standardize care.

◆ Quality Assessment

Quality assessment is the process of continuously striving to improve the delivery and outcome of care. It is a monitoring and evaluation feedback system aimed at capitalizing on opportunities to improve care and resolve patient care problems. The methods used to monitor care result in measurable and reliable data. Some examples of these methods include compliance to policy and procedures, audits, adherence to professionally recognized methods of determining patient perception of outcome and delivery of care, and appropriate use of resources.

A nursing leadership committee oversees quality assessment. The committee ensures that monitoring systems are in place, ongoing, and effective. The committee receives effectiveness reports from each nursing division or unit on a regular basis. The committee also examines and approves indicators and criteria for use in monitoring nursing care. Performance is measured to ensure safe, efficient, and effective care.

Monitoring nursing care includes reviewing physicians' orders, reporting and recording the application of nursing procedures and techniques, and patient teaching. Outcomes are interpreted in terms of the health-wellness state of a patient after receiving care. A monitoring study may be carried out several days before discharge. It facilitates prevention of problems, especially for the patient whose care is reviewed, and is helpful in the evaluation of day-to-day management of care.

Although there are various tools and types of methods designed for patient care, the purpose is the same: efficient, safe, and economical nursing care to every patient. This type of care meets the needs of the patient and promotes satisfaction in the giver and the receiver.

◆ *Study Helps*

1. Why must nursing care undergo changes?
2. Which personnel are included in nursing service today?
3. State and explain the role and functions of the registered nurse.
4. List the two types of student nurses and briefly state their functions.
5. How is licensure obtained?
6. What does the title LPN mean? What is the responsibility of the LPN?
7. Which types of assignments are given to nursing assistants?
8. State the differences between ward or unit clerks and unit managers.
9. How are nursing care assignments made?
10. What does functional patient care mean?
11. What is team nursing and how does it function?
12. What does progressive patient care involve?
13. When are same day surgery patients admitted and discharged?
14. What is included in a nursing care plan?
15. What is included in a nursing assessment?
16. List three community health services.
17. What is primary care nursing?
18. List the four components of the nursing process.
19. Define quality assessment.
20. What is the duty of the nursing leadership committee?

Bibliography

Christensen B, Kockrow E: *Foundations of nursing,* ed 1, St Louis, 1991, Mosby.
Cookfair JM: *Nursing process and practice in the community,* ed 1, St Louis, 1991, Mosby.
Deloughery G: *Issues and trends in nursing,* ed 1, St Louis, 1991, Mosby.

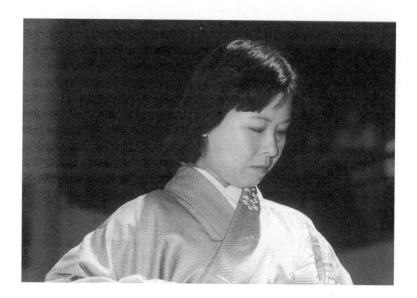

Objectives

At the completion of this chapter the student practical nurse will be able to:

- Identify the four ethnic-racial minorities.

- Summarize the spiritual needs of Catholics, Protestants, Jews, and persons in other denominations.

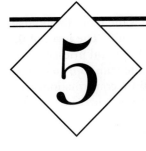

Religions, Culture, and Ethnic Groups

Total patient care includes not only the physical care that you give to your patients during their illness but also spiritual care encompassing all religious groups. In some institutions there are routine visits by various religious representatives.

On routine visits or when a religious representative is called to visit patients, you should extend every courtesy possible. Your assistance may be required; you must be understanding and helpful, regardless of your own religious affiliations. You must respect your patients' wishes, ensure privacy, understand their religious practices, and prepare necessary articles for these practices to be carried out.

Some patients who have been indifferent to religion may find it meaningful during illness. You are often the one who is asked to contact your patient's religious representatives; therefore one of your duties is to administer to your patient's spiritual needs.

The majority of Americans identify themselves as either Catholic, Protestant, or Jewish. Because of the variations in religions and the differences in a patient's attitudes toward them, you must handle each one differently. You must know each patient's religious attitudes before you can offer intelligent and helpful assistance. A brief account of each of the major faiths may help you to understand better the various beliefs and attitudes of your patients.

Because of the unique practices and customs of Catholic and Jewish patients in the hospital setting, necessary details are fully explained. These practices are founded on their beliefs. Therefore a knowledge and understanding of these beliefs must be obtained and understood to meet the patient's spiritual needs adequately.

◆ Major Religions

Catholicism

Those of the Catholic faith recognize that their religion began with the birth of Jesus Christ. They believe that Christ is God, who lived as a human, suffered, and died for the spiritual welfare of the human race.

The Roman Catholic Church traces its foundation to Peter, one of the twelve apostles chosen by Jesus to carry on His work after His death. Peter, as the first official head of the church, passed down this line of authority to the present pontiff. The head of the Roman Catholic Church is known as the *pope.* There are also bishops and priests, whose principal functions are to preach and minister to the people of the church by means of seven sacraments. The seven sacraments of this church are baptism, confirmation, Holy Eucharist (Communion), reconciliation (confession), Holy Orders, matrimony, and sacrament of the sick. The four sacraments that you as a practical nurse will most commonly encounter in meeting the spiritual needs of your Catholic patients are baptism, reconciliation, Holy Eucharist, and sacrament of the sick.

Any time a Catholic patient is admitted to the hospital, the priest should be notified so that he may visit the patient. Regard the priest's visit as a means of fulfilling the spiritual needs of your patient, not as a sign of danger or impending death. When a priest is needed, you should call him as soon as possible, regardless of the time and without any delay. It is most desirable for the patient's and the family's peace of mind that the priest arrive while the patient is still conscious if at all possible.

Baptism. Because the Catholic patient believes that baptism is absolutely necessary for salvation, any adult, child, or newborn, including a miscarriage of a living fetus, must be baptized, if not previously baptized, when in danger of death. This emergency baptism may be performed by anyone if a priest is not available. It is preferable to have a Catholic physician or nurse, if present, baptize the patient. If this is not practical or possible, you may and should baptize the patient, regardless of your religion. The only prerequisite for administering this sacrament is that you have the desire to carry out the religious beliefs of this patient's religion; then you must perform the procedure correctly. The sacrament is administered by pouring water over the forehead of the patient or, if this is not possible, over any skin surface and saying *at the same time* these words: "I baptize you in the Name of the Father and of the Son and of the Holy Spirit."

If you have any doubt as to whether the patient is still alive or has been baptized before, administer the sacrament conditionally. This is done by prefixing the baptismal words: "If you are capable of being baptized, I baptize you in the Name of the Father ...." By using the word *capable,* you include the facts that the patient is still alive, that he has the right disposition to receive the sacrament if he is an adult, and that he has never been baptized before. It is important to remember that the words must be said at the *same* time as you are pouring the water. The water must touch the skin itself, meaning that if there is any secretion, drainage, or foreign material on the skin, it must be cleansed before pouring the water. The hospital chaplain should be notified later that the emergency baptism was administered to the patient.

Mass. To attend Mass on Sundays and holy days of obligation is the first commandment of the Catholic Church. Catholics pay homage to God by their participation in the liturgy of the Mass, which is the central prayer of the Catholic religion. A person may have a legitimate excuse, such as illness or an emergency, for not attending Mass on Sundays or holy days.

In the hospital setting your patient may want to attend Mass in the hospital chapel if the hospital has one. If the patient's condition warrants attendance and permission of the attending physician has been obtained, assist your patient to the chapel either in a wheelchair or by walking, depending on his physical condition.

If unable to attend Mass, some patients like to read prayer books or recite prayers in the hospital room to fulfill this obligation. Some may desire to watch a televised Mass on Sunday mornings. In these cases you should give them adequate privacy.

It is a good point to remember that hospitalized patients are not obligated to attend Sunday Mass. The fact that they have been admitted to the hospital excuses them from this obligation. However, the patient's conscience, his physical condition, and the necessary medical permission should be the guiding factors in making this decision. A Catholic patient should never be forced to attend Sunday Mass or be judged for not attending this service.

Reconciliation. The sacrament of reconciliation is also referred to as *confession* or *penance.* In this sacrament Catholics seek reconciliation with God by expressing sorrow for their offenses against God or others. The priest offers a sign of this forgiveness through the words of absolution. It is advisable to ask Catholic patients if they would like to see a priest on admission to the hospital, before going to surgery, in case of an accident, or in any critical illness. Privacy should be ensured, and the priest should be provided with a chair so that he may talk with the patient. To a Catholic patient this sacrament may be a form of therapy as valuable as medication and treatment.

Holy Eucharist. Holy Eucharist, or Communion, is regarded as another important sacrament for the Catholic patient because he believes that he receives by way of bread and wine the Body and Blood, Soul and Divinity of Jesus Christ. Communion is usually received frequently but *must* be received during the Easter season. If possible, Communion is always given when there is danger of death and may be requested by the patient before going to the operating room.

A priest should be called any time a Catholic patient is in danger of death, regardless of whether he is a practicing Catholic. If the patient is capable of receiving Holy Communion, he may do so at this time.

Sacrament of the sick. The sacrament of the sick consists of anointment with holy oils. It is given to all those who have a serious illness or are facing serious surgery. Usually the priest and patient together make the decision; however, a priest should be called at the family's request or if the nurse sees a marked deterioration in the patient's condition. If a patient is unconscious, a priest should be called and given the details of the individual's condition.

Food practices. The rules of fasting and abstinence have been changed; fasting is now voluntary. Ash Wednesday and Good Friday are the only days requiring complete fasting and abstinence. However, you may discover some patients who prefer to follow the older practices. According to the older practice, fasting restricts persons between the ages of 21 and 60 to one full meal a day with limitations placed on the other meals. Abstinence restricts the use of meat for those 14 years of age or older every Friday, on ember days, and on other designated vigils.

Protestantism

Episcopalians, Methodists, Lutherans, Presbyterians, Baptists, members of the United Church of Christ, and Seventh-Day Adventists are classified as Protestants. Although these denominations have differences, they have many beliefs in common. These differences and beliefs are briefly noted.

Episcopalians. Episcopalians profess many of the Catholic beliefs but do not recognize the pope as Christ's vicar and head of the church. Private confession exists but is not compulsory. Episcopalians follow the Bible as a guide but do not hold to exact interpretation. They believe in heaven and hell but do not believe that heaven and hell exist as places. They make and observe laws concerning divorce and birth control. They use Holy Unction for those in danger of death but more often as a sacrament of healing. Episcopalian patients often like to receive Holy Communion. They believe baptism should be performed if an infant shows signs of dying.

Methodists. Methodists believe that religion is a personal matter. They believe that it is what a person feels. Conscience dictates their actions. They force changes when they believe changes are needed. The Methodist religion accepts baptism of all other denominations. They accept baptism by sprinkling or by immersion into water in either infancy or adulthood. They do not believe in canonization of saints or in purgatory. They believe that after death the good are rewarded and the evil are punished. They have flexible laws concerning divorce and birth control.

Lutherans. The Lutheran religion accepts the Trinity and regards Christ as both God and man. They believe that faith is the integral part of religion. Confirmation is considered a rite, not a sacrament, in their religion. Their practiced sacraments are baptism (by sprinkling for children and adults) and Communion. They believe that the presence of Christ is real in Communion.

Presbyterians. Presbyterians emphasize sovereignty of one God in three persons. They believe in the Bible and in heaven and hell. They believe that salvation cannot be obtained by living a good life because it is a gratuitous gift from God. They practice the sacraments of baptism (usually sprinkling) and Communion. They believe that Christ is present in spirit in Communion.

Baptists. Historically, Baptists are not Protestants because they existed as a denomination before the Reformation by Martin Luther. However, they are often classified as Protestants. The Baptists have no formal creed but emphasize that Christ heads the church. They restrict baptism to those old enough to understand its meaning. They practice total immersion. They take Communion as a remembrance of Christ's death. They often confess their sins openly before the congregation and ask forgiveness in this way. However, this method is not mandatory.

United Church of Christ. The United Church of Christ, the result of a union in 1957 of the Evangelical and Reformed Church and the Congregational Christian

Church, bases its beliefs and teachings on Holy Scripture. Practices include infant baptism, with full communicant church membership beginning at ages 12 to 14. The sacrament of the Lord's Supper is open to all Christian believers. Its policy is understanding of, respect for, and cooperation with all Christian groups.

Seventh-Day Adventists. The Seventh-Day Adventist religion is basically Protestant. Their members are usually vegetarians. They do not believe in infant baptism. This denomination believes in study and devotional readings of the Bible, individually and in groups. They believe in public and private worship emphasizing prayer. They require their members to carry out the teachings of the Bible as interpreted by the leaders of the churches and by the individual person.

Protestant Baptism. Baptism, as essential for salvation, is not the belief of some Protestant denominations. They believe in the right of the individual to choose the type of religion he believes meets his own needs in dealing with God. Certain institutions may be referred to as "ordinances in another religion."

A Protestant minister should be contacted anytime, day or night, if his presence is requested by the patient or by the patient's family. It is best if the minister arrives while the patient is still conscious or before he has received any sedation.

When a patient believes that baptism is essential to salvation and there is any doubt as to whether the minister will arrive in time, then you as a practical nurse may baptize an adult or child who has not been baptized. There must be a witness or sponsor present who should be another baptized person if possible. While baptizing the patient, the practical nurse must make sure the water touches the skin, while saying the words: "(The patient's name, if known), I baptize you in the Name of the Father and of the Son and of the Holy Spirit." The words must be said while the water is being poured on the forehead or, if this is impossible, any other part of the body.

Emergency baptism should be reported to the proper person so that the family may be notified that it was performed (if this is feasible). Baptism should be recorded on the patient's chart, in the nurse's notes, or on the admission sheet, as indicated by the policy of the hospital.

Other Denominations

Other denominations are not Catholic or Protestant. Some of these are Jehovah's Witnesses, Friends (Quakers), Christian Scientists, the Eastern Orthodox Church, and the Church of Jesus Christ of Latter-Day Saints. These denominations are briefly presented.

Jehovah's Witnesses. Jehovah's Witnesses stress one God (Jehovah). Their beliefs come from the Bible. The beliefs of these people prevent them from receiving whole blood, blood plasma, or any blood derivative.

Friends (Quakers). The Society of Friends (Quakers) has no ministers. Spiritual needs are met through members of the meeting. They have individual interpretations and practices.

Christian Scientists. Christian Scientists believe in spiritual healing. These patients are usually taken care of in one of their church-operated nursing homes or at home. If a Christian Scientist is admitted to a hospital because of an emergency, a Christian Science practitioner should be contacted. If a Christian Scientist is admitted to the hospital through a private physician, the written orders of the physician are to be followed.

Eastern Orthodox Church. Because the Eastern Orthodox Church has many of the same beliefs and practices as the Roman Catholic Church, it is wise to check to see which religious representative should be notified.

The Church of Jesus Christ of Latter-Day Saints (Mormons). This religion was organized by Joseph Smith in 1830. The Mormons believe in the Bible, as translated by the Mormon Church in the Book of Mormon, as the word of God; in the gifts of prophecy, healing, and revelation; and in the return of Christ to rule the earth in person. They practice the rites of baptism and the Lord's Supper. They maintain an extensive welfare program to assist needy members and support numerous missionaries overseas. In some cases of emergency the welfare recipients need not make repayment. Members of this religion do not believe in infant baptism. Their health laws do not allow tea, coffee, cola, alcohol, or tobacco. They do not believe in deathbed repentance but do believe in anointing the patient with olive oil before performing procedures and in asking a blessing for the patient.

Judaism

The Jewish religious year is based on a lunar calendar instead of the solar calendar. The Jewish faith is based on the five books of Moses, called the *Torah*. The Jewish religion follows the teachings of Moses. Today there are three types of Jewish groups. The Orthodox group is the oldest and the most resistant to ritualistic change. The Conservative group is less resistant to ritualistic change. The Reform group is the modern group that often makes deliberate changes in its ritual. The Jewish representative is known as the *rabbi*. He is the one to be contacted for a Jewish patient.

Sabbath. The Sabbath, observed from sunset Friday until after sunset Saturday, is a day for prayer, rest, and study. Services are held on Friday evenings and Saturday mornings. The Sabbath meal is an important observance. The family may have a lighting-of-candles ritual. This may be requested by some patients.

Food practices. Food practices vary according to whether the patient is Orthodox, Conservative, or Reformed. The "kosher" practice is observed by the Orthodox group, the Conservative group, and some Reformed Jews. In the kosher practice the main dietary laws involve utensils, meats, fish, and dairy products.

The utensils are kept in two separate groups; one group is used to prepare meat dishes and the other to prepare dishes containing dairy products. These utensils include dishes, silverware, and pans. When a set of glassware is used, it must be cleansed in a special way between uses.

Meat must come from divided-hoofed mammals such as cows, antelope, goats, and deer. These mammals must chew a cud. Other meats that may be eaten come from any fowl, such as turkeys, geese, and chickens, but must exclude any birds of prey. All meats must be slaughtered and prepared in a kosher way; all blood must be removed.

Fish that have both scales and fins do not come under the regulation of meat. They may be eaten with either dairy products or meat if they are prepared with a vegetable shortening.

Dairy products are not eaten with or after a meat meal. Eggs may be served with meat. Vegetables may be used as a substitute for meat.

Today many food products are manufactured in accordance with kosher dietary standards and these foods are marked with a XX. Foods marked as *pareve* (neither meat nor dairy product) may be served with meat or dairy products.

The *Kosher Products Directory* is published annually and may be obtained free from the Union of Orthodox Jewish Congregations of America.

When the physician believes that fasting would endanger the patient's life, the patient is excused from observing a fast.

Circumcision. Circumcision is a religious custom that takes place on the eighth day after birth unless contraindicated for medical reasons. This is a religious custom with prescribed rituals. At this time the boy receives his name. An obstetrician or surgeon may perform the circumcision on a Reformed Jew, with the rabbi reading certain prayers. Female children are named in their parents' house of worship, with the rabbi saying appropriate prayers.

Bar Mitzvah (boys), Bas Mitzvah (girls). Bar mitzvah and bas mitzvah are ceremonies celebrated after a boy's and girl's thirteenth birthday. These ceremonies signify religious maturity.

Jewish holidays. Some of the Jewish holidays are Rosh Hashanah, Yom Kippur, Succoth, Hanukkah, Passover, and Shavuoth.

Rosh Hashanah. Rosh Hashanah is a High Holiday; it is also the Jewish New Year. This is a day in autumn when God judges the deeds of man.

Yom Kippur. Yom Kippur is the Day of Atonement and is celebrated 10 days after the Jewish New Year. This holiday is celebrated by fasting and prayer and ends the penitence period.

Succoth. Succoth is similar to the solar calendar day of Thanksgiving. This holiday is celebrated for 9 days and ends with selected readings from Jewish scripture.

Hanukkah. Hanukkah falls near the solar calendar day of Christmas and is celebrated for 8 days with the lighting of candles.

Passover. Passover falls near the solar calendar day of Easter. This holiday is celebrated for 8 days with special foods (unleavened breads) and services.

Shavuoth. Shavuoth is celebrated in commemoration of receiving the Ten Commandments and may be confirmation day for Jewish adolescents.

Death procedures. Death procedures vary according to the three Jewish groups. The Orthodox and Conservative Jews do not believe in autopsies. They believe that a person near death should not be left alone. Even in the Reform group, members of the family and the rabbi usually stay with a dying person. The Orthodox and Conservative groups do not believe in embalming. Therefore, if possible, the funeral is held before sundown on the day the patient dies. They do not believe in burial on the Sabbath and certain holidays. They believe in sitting Shiva for 7 days after a death.

All these rules have been altered in the Reformed group to spare the feelings of the saddened family and to give support and consolation.

If no specific instructions as to the burial ceremonies have been received, then the body should be prepared according to hospital procedure.

Religion plays an important part in the lives of most people; therefore the spiritual leaders join the team of the hospital staff in meeting the patient's needs. As a practical nurse you should be familiar with the various religions so that you can carry through your important role in meeting the complete needs of your patients (see Table 5-1).

Table 5-1 ◇ Summary of religious rites and practices

Jewish	Protestant	Roman Catholic
Death and autopsy		
Family or rabbi will make arrangements for burial	Most Protestant denominations administer last sacraments, if they believe in them, before death occurs	Roman Catholics should receive, if possible and desirable, sacrament of the sick, penance, and Holy Eucharist
Because some Jews object to autopsy, consult rabbi or family regarding autopsy	No moral objection to autopsy	Ritual should be performed during illness or before death
		No moral objection to autopsy
Conditions involving serious illnesses		
May not desire surgical procedure performed on Sabbath or holy day	May desire to see minister to pray and talk	When ill or in danger of death, may desire to receive penance, Holy Communion, and sacrament of the sick
May desire to see rabbi	Minister determines whether patient is to receive Holy Communion, confession, or Extreme Unction	Chaplain or parish priest administers sacraments as determined by condition and desire of patient

◆ Culture

Culture is the customary beliefs, material traits, and social forms of a religious, racial, or social group. Recognition of cultural differences is important in understanding the behavior of ourselves and others. Culture refers to human activities that are passed from one generation to the next. It applies to the collective ways of life in a group of people. It includes some basics such as language, diet, family support groups, religion, mating, government, wars, clothing, shelter, and daily life. No two cultures are exactly alike, although most have similar fundamental needs. The cultural characteristics of a group may or may not be exhibited by every individual in that group.

Subcultures are fairly large numbers of people, who, although members of a larger cultural group, have shared characteristics that are not common to all members of the culture. For example, because of their knowledge and skills, practical nurses belong to a subculture.

◆ Ethnic Groups

Ethnicity refers to races or large groups of people classed according to common traits and customs. In the United States, ethnic groups are based on the following factors: religion, race, language, politics, and nationality. These factors differentiate minority groups in our society.

Because you are human, you may be affected by the prejudices of others. You may even have some prejudices of your own. Acceptance of the fact that all persons are created equal, regardless of their race, may help you to overcome prejudices and better meet your patient's needs.

Race has become difficult to classify because of mobility, intermarriage, and intermixing of cultures, which blend races so that no line can be drawn between any two of them. Humans have been divided into the following three major races by some anthropologists:

1. Mongolian race, which is made up of most of the people of the Far East, such as the Japanese and Chinese
2. Negro or black race, which is made up of most dark-skinned people, such as those of African descent
3. Caucasian or white race, which is made up of light-skinned people who share certain physical features, such as most people from Europe, the Middle East, and part of the East Indies

You may hear groups called the "Jewish race" or the "American race," but these are incorrect. These groups are not races but a religious group and a national group, respectively.

The distinguishing characteristics of races are minor physical differences such as skin color, facial features, and body size. The changes have probably come about through a natural process of evolution in which individuals have changed to adjust to their environmental conditions. Physical differences are the only ones that can be found. The main racial stocks have been mixing so that no definite line can be drawn between any two races. No race is better or more intelligent than another. Given equal social, educational, economic, and environmental backgrounds, each race can parallel the achievements of the other races.

Proof of this statement is found in the life of Mary Eliza Mahoney, the first black nursing graduate. From a class of forty, only three students graduated in 1879 from the 16-month course given at the New England Hospital for Women and Children. Mahoney was one of the three graduates and the only black student in her class. Her fine record at school, skill, devotion, and intelligence in pursuing her nursing vocation in Boston after graduation furthered intergroup relationships and paved the way for blacks to achieve a place in nursing.

In 1909 she gave the welcoming address at the first conference of the National Association of Colored Graduate Nurses. In 1936 this Association initiated the Mary Mahoney Medal in her honor. The medal serves as a symbol of the opportunities in nursing for individuals of all races, creeds, and nationalities.

As a nurse you are responsible for your patient's well-being, regardless of his race, nationality, or religion. Every person has rights. You should never be convinced by anyone that this is not true. You must safeguard the patient's rights, regardless of your feelings or those of others, for all humans are equal.

◆ *Study Helps*

1. Why is it necessary to know and understand the religious beliefs of your patients?
2. What are the beliefs of the Catholic religion?
3. How would you meet the spiritual needs of a critically ill or dying Catholic patient?
4. How is conditional baptism administered?
5. Why is the Holy Eucharist so important to the Catholic patient?
6. What are the current regulations with regard to fasting and abstinence for the modern-day Catholic?
7. Which denominations are classified under Protestantism? Briefly describe each denomination's beliefs and practices.
8. What is the basis of the Jewish religion? What are its religious practices and customs?
9. Who was the first black nurse?
10. What does the Mary Mahoney Medal symbolize?
11. Define *culture*.

Bibliography

Collins M: *Communications in health care,* ed 2, St. Louis, 1983, Mosby.
Cox ML: Notes from the chairperson, *Council on intercultural nursing newsletter* 1:1, 1981.
Orque MS, Bloch B, Monrroy LSA: *Ethnic nursing care,* St Louis, 1983, Mosby.
Primeaux M, Henderson G: *Transcultural health care,* Reading, Mass, 1981, Addison-Wesley.
Saxton DF, Nugent PM, Pelikan PK: *Mosby's comprehensive review of nursing,* ed 13, St Louis, 1990, Mosby.
Smith H: *The religions of man,* New York, 1961, Mentor Books.
Yannes-Eyles M: *Mosby's comprehensive review of practical nursing,* ed 11, St Louis, 1994, Mosby.

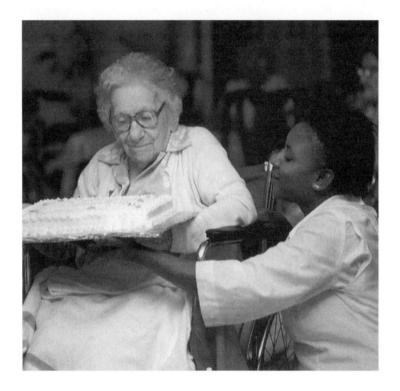

Objectives

At the completion of this chapter the student practical nurse will be able to:

♦ Describe the five stages of dying.

♦ Describe your role as a nurse in dealing with the patient's visitors and family.

♦ Identify specific needs of abortion, child abuse, elderly, mentally ill, and suit-prone patients.

6 Dealing With Patients Who Have Special Needs

As a student practical nurse and later as a licensed practical nurse, you will be confronted with various types of patient needs. The manner in which you handle these needs is determined by your understanding of the need, the patient involved, the type of training you have received, and your own personal makeup. Your reactions to situations may vary from those of others. The level of maturity you have acquired is an important factor determining your reactions. However, a clear knowledge and understanding of common needs are assets when you are confronted with them. A few of the common needs are discussed in this chapter.

◆ Death

Death is a biological process that occurs at the end of life. When death occurs, all vital body functions cease. A human is born, lives a designated life-span, and dies as the result of the termination of this life-span. This is true of every living organism. The exact length of the human life-span is unknown to anyone. Certain factors play an important role in its termination. Some of these are disease conditions, mental disturbances, accidents, and old age. By the laws of nature every human must die. However, few people are prepared or ready to die. Death is often difficult to accept, both for the patient who is facing death and for the family members who must suffer separation from their loved one.

Every individual develops a concept of death. To young children, death is like sleep. It has no finality. They do not associate death with themselves. They do not regard it as something that happens to everyone. By 9 or 10 years of age, children regard death as inevitable. To them everyone lives and then dies. The adolescent regards death as a mystery and ponders an afterlife, and as a teenager he associates death with romance and self-sacrifice. Young adults love life. They think of death as the termination of all things and may display hostile feelings toward it. The middle-aged person is very aware of death. In this age group, illnesses may place emphasis on the possibility of dying. Older persons often discuss death with their clergyman. They appear to be the most prepared to face death; however, there are stages that all patients pass through before accepting death. These stages are denial, anger, bargaining, depression, and acceptance.

Denial is the stage in which the patient refuses to believe he is going to die. This is a temporary defense that exists in all persons at some time.

Anger is directed at everyone and everything. It is difficult for the nursing staff to manage because it may explode in any direction. You should support the patient in his efforts to make day-by-day decisions.

Bargaining means that the patient wants an extension of time so that he may see someone, do one last task, or wait until some event is passed such as a birth. If possible you should rearrange treatments or visiting hours to try to fulfill the expressed needs of the dying person.

Depression is the preparatory grief stage. The dying person is sad and may withdraw from his family and the staff. At this time his wishes must take precedence over everyone else's.

Acceptance is the prelude to a peaceful death. During this stage the patient may be tired and weak and may doze frequently. However, you should be aware of his loneliness and not abandon him in his dying stage. Some patients never attain acceptance and fight to the end. You have to react to their behavior as it occurs and offer emotional support by being present and listening.

To be of assistance to the dying patient, his relatives, and friends, you must be aware of your own feelings toward death and analyze these feelings. Your approach to death must be realistic. Just as everything you use wears out at some time, so does the human body. Sometimes because of excessive use or faulty mechanism, the equipment may have a short life-span. Prolonged use or congenital malformation of organs of the body may shorten the life-span. A healthy appearance does not necessarily mean that all body structures are functioning correctly. All structures have a specific purpose. If one becomes defective, the entire body is affected.

It is difficult to understand that the effect of disease on the body often ends in death. The more difficult situations to understand are deaths that occur as a result of mental disturbances and accidents. Suicide is the taking of one's own life. It is usually caused by a highly charged emotional situation or depressed state. The person who takes his own life may not be considered responsible for this act.

Accidents cause many deaths each year. They may result from carelessness or merely from strange causes or circumstances. This type of death is difficult to accept because it is so sudden; usually involves healthy individuals, many of whom are young; and produces a state of shock in the surviving relatives. Many emotions are elicited by accidental deaths. Unfairness, cruelty, despair, loss, and rebellion are common emotions displayed. Relatives and friends may feel that God has been unjust to them and to their families. They may begin to wonder if there is a God. If there is, then how could He be so cruel as to allow this to happen? They may rebel against Him and against society. They may become embittered. For a time they may feel that life is not worth living if they must live it without their loved one. But life continues, and the bereaved persons must adjust themselves and their lives to meet this present loss. Some may need help adjusting.

Persons who believe in an afterlife often find death easier to accept than those who do not. They regard death as a temporary separation. They think of it as a state of complete happiness and bliss. They feel relieved that the period of suffering is ended for their loved one. Some feel that the loved one's real purpose in life has been accomplished. They regard life as a journey leading to eternal life, which is a permanent resting place, a place in which all their hopes and desires are fulfilled. Some think of it as heaven, where the deceased person is enjoying the company of God.

Religious training plays an important part in determining a person's particular feelings about and attitude toward death. You should know the religion of the dying patient and his family to be of real assistance to them in their time of need.

Patient's Feelings

Few persons are ever ready to die. The patient often experiences real fear when death is approaching. He is afraid of the unknown. If he does not believe in an afterlife, then life is terminating with real finality. To this patient death means a complete separation forever from friends and relatives. It means the end of everything. This type of patient clings to every last shred of life.

Patients who believe in an eternity also suffer from uncertainty and fear. They may fear the judgment of God. The Catholic patient may fear condemnation to purgatory or hell for all eternity. Those who regard death as a journey often manifest a degree of peace. However, they still fear the uncertainty of the future.

How should you deal with the dying patient? First of all, know his religion and notify his clergyman if so desired or necessary. Remain with the dying patient if possible. No one wants to die alone. Pray with him, if requested or indicated. Let the patient know that you are there. This can be done by holding his hand, stroking his arm or face, or speaking softly to him. Render the necessary nursing care to afford him comfort. Never speak in his presence as though he were already dead or incapable of hearing what you are saying. The last sense to disappear in a dying patient is that of hearing. He often hears more than you think possible in his condition. If the patient knows that those who care for him are with him, this brings tranquility and peace to him. He feels safe as long as his loved ones are with him. Everyone is afraid of the unknown. However, when it is necessary to venture into it, it gives the frightened person courage to know that someone is with him.

Family's Reaction

The family of a dying patient may react in various ways. They may be emotional almost to the point of hysteria. They may be inconsolable at this time. The best response is to get the family involved in some type of activity. Involvement may take the form of notifying other members of the family or making certain arrangements when death becomes inevitable. The physician may order a sedative to calm a relative. If the relatives are causing a disturbance in the dying patient's room or in the corridor, you should take them to an enclosed waiting room or any other private place. Remain with them until they have composed themselves. This type of behavior may be upsetting to the dying patient as well as to the other patients in the unit.

Some relatives react in a hostile manner. They may blame the physician or the hospital or both for the person's death. They often say things that they ordinarily do not feel and would not say if they were not emotionally upset. This type of behavior may be irritating to hospital personnel. However, the best manner in which to check these feelings of hostility or resentment is to show kindness and understanding.

The most difficult situation with which you may have to cope is the family who does not react at all. They appear relieved over the possibility of the approaching death of their relative. Their relief is for themselves, not for the patient. They may be interested in the monetary possessions that they have planned to inherit. They are often greedy and stop at nothing to get what they want. Your normal reaction to this type of situation may be disgust and perhaps hatred. You may wonder how anyone could be so cruel or callous. You are inclined to protect the patient from them. In many cases the dying person has long been aware of his relatives' feelings toward him. This awareness may hurt him and make him feel completely alone. Your greatest service is to remain with the patient and show him that you care about him as a person. He needs someone to be kind to him. In all probability, you will have little effect on the relatives. As a professional person you must always show tolerance and kindness. Your conduct stands as a monument to your profession. It may have a lasting effect on the relatives although it may not be apparent at the time.

Coping With the Situation

Regardless of which reactions the family may portray, there are certain things that must be done. Everything possible must be done to prevent other patients from becoming upset over the death of another patient. This is accomplished by closing the other patients' doors and especially the door to the room of the dying or dead patient. Working in a quiet, efficient manner minimizes the attention drawn to this area. Upset relatives may be isolated in a closed waiting room.

Relatives may ask many questions after their loved one's death. If you listen and show that you are interested and concerned, this may be really all they want of you. If they talk long enough, they usually solve their own problems and answer their own questions. Try listening rather than answering in situations such as these. The family must come to its own decisions regarding funeral arrangements and burial. They must decide whether they wish for a postmortem examination. If they ask your advice concerning an autopsy, you may explain the meaning of an autopsy to them in simple terms. An example may be: "An autopsy is similar to a surgical operation. The abdomen and sometimes the head are opened, and the organs are examined." You may state the advantages of having an autopsy performed. These advantages include determining the real cause of death, perhaps helping another member of the family who may at some future date have similar symptoms, and helping to increase medical knowledge through this careful and educational procedure. Assure the family that if they do desire this examination, the dead patient will not be disfigured in any way. The family should never be forced into this decision. Usually the physician or house physician seeks this permission. Nevertheless, you may be the person from whom the relatives seek advice. Always refer them to their physician for anything other than a simple explanation.

If the family is indecisive and knows no funeral director, you may direct them to the yellow pages of the telephone directory. The choice should be left to them, and you should not influence them in making it. They can note the various locations and select one that is closest or most suitable to them.

Immediately after the patient has been pronounced dead, the family should be left alone with the deceased, if desired. This privacy should be allowed them. These last few minutes are greatly treasured. It also helps them to accept to some degree their loss and gives them the time needed to compose themselves.

While the body is being prepared, the family should be taken to a quiet, private place where they may discuss the necessary arrangements that must be made. In most hospitals the funeral director must be contacted and a release of the body to the undertaker must be signed before the family is permitted to leave.

The personal belongings of the deceased should be carefully packaged. Valuables should be personally given to a close member of the family, and a note should be made to this effect on the patient's chart. If you are uncertain as to which belongings are the patient's, you may ask a member of the family to help you gather the possessions. After all arrangements have been made and the necessary forms signed as required by the hospital, accompany the relatives to the exit.

After the relatives have departed, the body may be taken to the morgue. The chart must be completed. Use the procedure indicated by the hospital in which you are working.

If religion plays an important part in the burial arrangement and the family members have questions as to whom to contact, refer them to the hospital chaplain, their parish priest, or their minister. These persons can give them the necessary information they are seeking and direct them in these matters.

Death is personal to the bereaved relatives. The kindness and sympathy that you manifest to them are often remembered for a long time. You should be helpful to them, but they must make their own decisions. You must control your own emotions if you are to be of assistance to the family. They expect you to be the professional person that your vocation demands at all times.

◆ Single Mother

The single mother is faced with complex problems. She has the problem of being pregnant, plus the problem of not being accepted by society. In dealing with the single mother the best and most helpful attitude to maintain is that she is not a "bad girl" but a pregnant woman. Your attitude should be neither patronizing nor condescending. A single mother cannot be stereotyped. She may be from a wealthy family or a poor family. She may be of any race. She may be brilliant or dull, innocent or hardened. Regardless of her background, the single mother has real needs. She needs to receive proper medical attention for the existing pregnancy and counseling to help her face reality and make the necessary decisions that arise as a result of her pregnancy.

Where can she receive help? For the single mother who is still in high school or college, the school counseling service can give her the assistance she needs. For the single mother not in school many social service organizations offering this type of help run notices in the newspaper. They are also listed in the telephone directory. Not only do these organizations help provide counseling service, they also help obtain the necessary medical attention that is required and provide means for livelihood, food, and shelter.

The single mother faces many adjustments. Sometimes she is completely rejected by family and friends.

Homes for single mothers usually have work routines, counseling, rest periods, recreation, and infant care classes for those keeping their babies. These women receive prenatal care, including a balanced diet. They are admitted to the hospital for the delivery of their babies. After delivery they are assisted in completing forms for adoption if desired or in making living arrangements and finding employment.

Attitudes are changing regarding the single mother. Many couples who do not believe in traditional marriages are having planned children who are being reared by a single parent. Today more parents are beginning to accept responsibility for a daughter in this situation, allowing her to remain at home during the pregnancy. Single motherhood still presents an emotional situation to which the unmarried mother, family, friends, and society must adjust. Professional counseling assists the girl and her family.

Professional counseling is offered to the single mother by various agencies. This type of service should never be forced on anyone; it should be a personal choice and decision. The function of such counseling services is to help the mother establish herself as an individual, accept herself as she is, and make plans for the future.

A major decision for the single mother is whether to keep the baby or put it up for adoption. Neither adoption nor keeping the infant should be urged or insisted on. The mother must make the decision; however, she must be given both alternatives so that these may be explored in an unhurried manner.

The woman must adjust to the pregnancy itself. This adjustment involves physical and emotional factors. She may suffer from physical symptoms such as morning sickness or a feeling of distressing fullness. General mood swings also occur. At the beginning of the pregnancy she may have mixed feelings of elation and depression because of the physiological adjustment of her body to pregnancy. As the pregnancy progresses, the mother may be thrilled and awed with the impending birth of the child she has nourished and helped to form, or she may feel guilt and shame.

The period after delivery may be extremely difficult for the single mother who has decided to have her baby adopted. It is the policy of many organizations to show the baby to the mother one time only. It may create an emotional crisis for the mother to give her baby to someone else. This is the reason that professional counseling is continued after delivery until the mother has made satisfactory adjustment to postpartum life.

The adjustments of the single mother are numerous and difficult; she does not need or desire punishment, lectures, or censure but rather love, understanding, and hope. She should be treated with respect and dignity and not spoken about in whispered tones that tend to portray her as being "different" from other pregnant women. Be considerate but not patronizing.

◆ Abortion Patient

Since the 1973 decision of the Supreme Court a pregnancy may be terminated at the request of the woman. Interpretations of the decision vary from state to state and institution to institution with many changes made at all levels.

Many factors are involved with abortion, including medical, legal, religious, emotional, social, and family factors with which you must deal in a compassionate way.

With changes of abortion laws in the United States and abortions being performed legally, you have to take a close look at your own attitudes and feelings. The abortion patient requires understanding, kindness, and psychological support as well as regular nursing care to meet her needs. If you feel you are unable to meet the patient's total needs, discuss this honestly with your instructor, who can help you to cope with the situation in a realistic and mature manner. Employers have a right to know your beliefs regarding abortion and sterilization.

◆ Hostile, Aggressive Patient

In this chapter the hostile, aggressive patient is one whose activities are forward and exceed normal standards as a result of a driving inner force and excessive energy. The activities are willful acts that are contrary to acceptable standards of behavior.

The hostile, aggressive patient may become a real problem on a general nursing division. At first glance it may be difficult to understand the actions of this type of patient. It is easy to forget that sickness sometimes brings with it regression to former stages of development that may vary with the individual patient. A patient's defenses are down when he is ill. He often expresses his true self at a time like this. Emotions that have been suppressed find a release in some form.

Often the hostile, aggressive patient has had a strict childhood background. As a child he may have developed fears because of training that was harsh, prematurely instituted, and sometimes exaggerated. This type of control may have extended itself to an inhibition of even normal, healthy activity. Initiative may have been blocked. Spontaneity has often been sacrificed, and continuous defensive efforts must be made to judge authority figures and their wishes. Such a child becomes a "little angel," overly good, essentially timid, and noncontributing. He may have been forced to repress his anger. As a result this repressed hostility has grown until rigid defenses are needed now to control it. When a patient finds himself in a position in which his defenses are weakened, some of this repressed hostility may manifest itself in one or more of these symptoms: severe constipation, diarrhea, sleep disturbances, enuresis, or sexual advances.

The most threatening and difficult situation that may confront the female practical nurse may be advances made by the aggressive male patient. These advances are frightening because the female nurse is unsure of how to cope with them. She regards them as frightening and improper. By all means they are to be discouraged and dealt with adequately. A few suggestions may be helpful for the nurse who is ever confronted with this type of situation.

Always be in control of the situation. Act according to professional decorum. Do not let the patient know that you fear him. Accept the situation as a normal occurrence but one that you neither tolerate nor accept. If the advances are made verbally, change the subject. If this diversion fails, then state in a quiet but emphatic voice that you do not enjoy this type of conversation. If the patient continues despite your admonition, leave the room as soon as possible and report the incident to the team leader or head nurse.

If the advances are made by physical contact, such as grabbing your hand, trying to kiss you, or attempting to touch certain areas of your body, try to withdraw from the patient. If it is impossible because of the force he is exerting, tell him to stop this type of behavior immediately. Also, tell him that the incident will be reported to the hospital authorities. The patient must be made to realize that this behavior is inappropriate and that you as a professional person do not tolerate it. This may be referred to as *molestation,* which is a violation of a person's rights.

Molestation is the touching of another person's body without consent. A nurse does touch the body of a patient in the performance of duties. However, when a patient signs himself into the hospital, he gives the hospital and those caring for him permission to perform whatever duties are necessary. Therefore the nurse functions under this implied permission of the patient and is not guilty of molestation. The patient does not have any type of permission to touch the body of the nurse, and you as a nurse should not allow this in any form.

In nursing a belligerent patient differs from an aggressive, hostile patient in that he is combative and may show violence in words or actions. Additional help is usually supplied when rendering care to a patient in this condition. This type of behavior is often demonstrated by the alcoholic or emotionally disturbed patient.

◆ Shy, Withdrawn Patient

The shy, withdrawn patient is one who is quiet and does not express his feelings. This type of person often has a weak personality. He is excessively timid and afraid to mix with others. He may have demanded from his parents or his marriage partner an excessive amount of protection. He usually lacks the moral courage to stand up to a difficult situation. This type of patient tends to accept any illness that may develop and is frequently in a state of mental and physical weakness. He easily accepts defeat and becomes apathetic. He often shows no desire to recover because recovering involves the responsibility of returning to normal life. He avoids anxiety-producing situations. As a patient he must be coaxed, or at least encouraged, to eat, take medicine, or make any attempt to recover adequately. He usually does what he is told but nothing more. This patient needs understanding, sympathy, and friendly encouragement. This regard gives him a feeling of trust and confidence in you as a nurse and also gives him the incentive to help himself.

If a patient is prone to this type of behavior, hospitalization may exaggerate these symptoms. Hospitalization is a frightening experience to many patients. They feel insecure and are uncertain about the outcome of their illness. They are often afraid to express their feelings because they fear ridicule from their families and the hospital staff. They must be encouraged to express their feelings. If they feel that they can trust you, they will communicate their feelings either in words or in actions. They must be helped to accept their true roles as individual persons and as members of society.

◆ Drug Abuse Patient

Drug abuse, particularly among the young, is a big problem today. Drug abuse is not confined to urban ghetto areas. Affluent suburbia and rural communities are equally troubled. Members of all age groups abuse drugs. Drug use has now spread from college students to high school and junior high school students as "the thing to do."

There are many and varied programs available to the addict. With the increasing awareness of substance abuse as a health problem and less social stigma, more individuals are now seeking help. With this increase in knowledge more programs are available. Prevention programs such as health clinics and schools are available in community health settings. Care units offer inpatient, partial hospitalization, and day and evening outpatient programs. Psychologically the aim is toward control of self.

You must observe the drug abuse patient carefully for signs of withdrawal or evidence that drugs are being obtained from inside or outside the hospital. He may attempt to hide pills, especially during the early phase of withdrawal. The addict needs extra support; therefore your role is one of support and nonjudgmental participation.

◆ Alcoholic Patient

Alcoholism is an illness not peculiar to any particular kind of person. It affects people regardless of residence, age, sex, political affiliation, intelligence, social position, color, wealth, or occupation.

Alcohol is the most widely abused drug. In the United States, out of 10 million problem drinkers 6 million are estimated to be alcoholic. At the present, male alcoholics outnumber females about 5:1, but this ratio is decreasing. Although men appear to have more drinking problems in their twenties, women most frequently are in their thirties or forties. Alcoholism also affects the elderly population, perhaps as many as 90%. Although alcoholic treatment programs have been established for men for several years, a growing awareness of the problem in women is reshaping rehabilitation programs to include women's needs. As a student practical nurse you may come in contact with an alcoholic patient of any age and in any of the nursing divisions, including pediatrics.

Some characteristics of an alcoholic patient are denial, impulsiveness, evasion, projection, low frustration tolerance, ambivalence, manipulation, remorse, and low self-esteem. This list is not all inclusive, and not all alcoholics display all of these characteristics. If you recognize and accept such behavior as a part of your patient's alcoholism, you can better meet your responsibilities in giving total patient care.

Denial

The alcoholic almost always has difficulty in recognizing drinking or alcoholism as a problem. Although it may be perfectly clear to you, your patient's family, and many other people, your patient may not believe that this is really a problem.

Impulsiveness

The alcoholic often does things on the spur of the moment, without considering the outcome of the actions. The alcoholic is capable of understanding the results of his actions but does not or cannot take the time to consider these actions before he acts, such as when taking the first drink.

Evasion

The alcoholic hides drinking and tries to avoid any reference to it. The alcoholic talks about the weather, financial difficulties, or family problems in an effort to stay as far away as possible from discussing the matter of drinking.

Projection

The alcoholic generally attempts to rely heavily on the protective method of blaming his drinking problem on other people or circumstances. The alcoholic sees someone else as being responsible for the difficulty. For example, if the other person would change, then there would be no alcoholic problem.

Low Frustration Tolerance

Little things seem to upset the alcoholic more than they upset other people. The alcoholic seems unusually sensitive to criticism, anger, or other situations that other people would not notice.

Ambivalence

The alcoholic is extremely torn between not drinking and getting another drink. The alcoholic must be given every opportunity to recognize this ambivalence. If you are intolerant of either abstinence or drinking, you deprive the alcoholic of the opportunity to understand himself as completely as possible.

Manipulation

The alcoholic is a master at manipulating people and situations to his own advantage. The alcoholic frequently gets people to make special arrangements for him, vouch for him, protect him, or take some risk for him. After these things have been done for an alcoholic, the alcoholic frequently starts drinking again.

Remorse

The alcoholic experiences a great deal of remorse; sometimes it is so great that the alcoholic can no longer live with it and must have another drink. Increasing the remorse of an alcoholic by shaming, scolding, or belittling serves only to intensify the problem.

Low Self-Esteem

Perhaps the most overlooked characteristic of the alcoholic is his low self-esteem. Low self-esteem often goes unrecognized because it is masked by an air of confidence ("I can do anything; I have money, friends, and influence") that is exhibited by the alcoholic. Because he has fooled others for so long, it is difficult for the alcoholic to recognize low self-esteem.

◇   ◇   ◇

You should be aware of the treatment plan your alcoholic patient's physician has prescribed and reinforce and support your patient and his family in following this plan, whether it be referral to a rehabilitation center or to Alcoholics Anonymous.

◆ Child Abuse Patient

Child abuse or neglect is a serious and complex behavior problem. In all states, the Virgin Islands, and the District of Columbia, hospitals or other health care providers are now legally responsible for reporting suspected cases of child abuse. Child abuse or neglect should not be ruled out when a child is seen with long bone fractures, burns, bruises, scars, welts, cranial trauma, old fractures, or starvation. Further investigation is warranted in many of these cases.

The details of procedure and substance for reporting abuse or neglect may vary slightly from one state to another. Information needed to investigate child abuse usually includes name, age, address, persons responsible for the care of the child, and the nature and extent of the possible abuse.

As a student practical nurse, if you observe a child in the emergency room or the pediatric unit and suspect child neglect or abuse, you should immediately notify your instructor.

◆ Suit-Prone Patient

The suit-prone patient is usually a person who is generally unhappy and dissatisfied with all parts of life and therefore is more likely than any other type of patient to bring suit for malpractice when something goes wrong.

Because of the general public's awareness of the legal responsibilities of the physician, nurse, and hospital, lawsuits are brought much more readily for real or imagined negligence. Therefore you must know how to prevent malpractice claims.

Some warning signs to watch for and report to your instructor are the patient's questioning everything, complaining constantly, openly expressing hostility to his nurses or health care givers, asking names, taking notes of what his doctors and nurses say, and requesting his chart when discharged.

Most nursing malpractice suits are caused by the patient's dissatisfaction with care. Using good nursing practice, based on sound knowledge and skill, and acting as a reasonably prudent person under similar circumstances makes you less likely to be involved in a lawsuit. If you assess the individual's total needs, listen to the individual, and explain your actions, the patient will probably accept the care. If you are aware of a suit-prone patient, alert coworkers, keep accurate records, and notify your instructor, who can assist you in dealing with this type of patient.

◆ Elderly Patient

In 1935 the special needs of the elderly became publicly acknowledged with the introduction of Social Security. Retirement was forced on many economically unprepared older persons, leaving them with little hope for the future. As a result many persons had to live on a fixed income, which did not change as prices rose. This created needs in areas such as obtaining food, paying utility costs, finding adequate living quarters, and providing coverage for medical care.

Physical changes and the health needs of aging affect all aspects of the older person's life. The frequent feelings of loneliness, indecision, insecurity, helplessness, confusion, and rejection, as well as mental deterioration, must be considered. The physiological changes of aging may include impairment of the senses with maladjustment. The aging person's response and reaction time may be slowed. These changes may make it difficult to solve problems and carry out everyday activities. Whether the source of changes is physical, physiological, or sociological, the whole person responds to the changes.

The field of geriatrics is now considered a specialty. A Division for Geriatric Nursing was included in the 1966 American Nurses Association convention. This was important because now nursing recognizes that the elderly have the same health care needs as do people of other age-groups. As a gerontological nurse it is important to assist the older person to identify unmet needs and the resources for meeting those needs. Although personal independence is to be encouraged, as a student nurse you must be aware of the normal changes brought about by the aging process. Using patience you must help the patient to maintain dignity by resuming as active a life as possible.

New technologies are being developed that may lessen some needs of the elderly and may greatly increase their level of activity. Some of the technological achievements are better eyesight—with the use of lasers a cataract can be removed in minutes; better hearing—with improved hearing aids and implants; better memory—researchers are discovering new ways to restore memory; and less fear of approaching death—with thanatology (the study of death), people are learning ways to cope with death. Not only curing physical and mental ailments helps the elderly; improved television programs also help. Large screens help those with eyesight loss, subtitles help those with hearing loss, and remote control helps those who cannot leave their bed or chair. These improvements bring sports, movies, and current events into the home for the elderly to enjoy.

Some surveys have shown that by the year 2080 the number of Americans 85 years or older is expected to be 18.7 million. White women have the longest life expectancy, followed by black women. As our aging population increases, we must assume a leadership role in changing society's attitudes about the elderly so they can obtain a higher quality of life.

◆ Elderly Abused Patient

The elderly are suffering abuses such as neglect, physical assault, threats, and financial losses. Many are left in bed with soiled linens and clothes. They may have bruises that are said to be from falls. Families may threaten them with being placed in nursing homes, so the elderly usually remain quiet about being abused.

The abuse frequently comes from a son, daughter, or spouse, which may make elderly persons ashamed to tell that their own family could do such a thing. It is harder to recognize abuse in elderly persons because they are unable to be out in the community where they can be seen. Abuses and neglect may occur in institutions in the form of not keeping elderly persons and their surroundings clean, inadequate food, and rough treatment by the workers. Elderly persons frequently remain silent because they feel they have no other place to go.

The elderly abuse issue is now starting to be addressed by most state legislatures, universities, and conferences. Speakers are available in some areas to address elderly abuse. State laws vary as to the reporting of elderly abuse. Be familiar with the laws of your state.

As a student practical nurse who observes an elderly person and suspects neglect or abuse, you should report to your instructor, who can advise you what sources are available in your area to help the elderly.

◆ Chronic Pain Patient

Pain is a state in which the person reports discomfort or an uncomfortable sensation. Each person perceives and describes pain individually. Chronic pain is persistent or intermittent pain that lasts for a long time (usually for longer than 6 months). Chronic pain may be permanent, accompanied by residual disability, and caused by irreversible pathologic changes. The person experiencing chronic pain usually requires long periods of health care. Chronic pain is a constant companion. It is present 24 hours a day, 7 days a week. If pain is not present, the person questions why it is not or fears his actions will cause the pain to recur.

Chronic pain may severely impair the quality of life. It usually limits the mobility and function of a person. The chronic pain sufferer must live differently from the way he lived before his symptoms. Pain has to be considered with any other activities. Movement may present multiple problems. Dressing and undressing when desired may be a luxury that is not affordable because the movement necessary to carry out usual activities may generate unbearable pain. Thus chronic pain may limit the amount and way the person performs his daily personal care activities. Holding a job and engaging in social activities may not be possible because of the unpredictable return of pain or the amount of pain caused by the activity.

The course of chronic pain is unpredictable. One day a person may feel better and think he will continue to improve, only to experience an increase in discomfort the very next day. Sometimes he is able to decide what caused the increase in pain and at other times he cannot identify the cause.

Pain is also fatiguing. Much energy is necessary to deal with pain. It also disturbs sleep. When an individual is uncomfortable, it is difficult to sleep. When other distractions and activities are absent, it also seems that the person focuses on the pain he is experiencing. When a person with chronic pain complains of feeling fatigued, realize that this is true.

The person with chronic pain often has to depend on others for his care. It is difficult to have someone else do actions he is used to doing for himself. Because of the pain, fatigue, and adjusting to a different life-style, a person often becomes irritable. Unfortunately the persons most likely to have to deal with his irritability are the ones closest to him—his family and the nurses.

Nurses, doctors, and lay persons tend to prefer not to interact with people with chronic pain. They prefer persons who are going to be experiencing pain for a limited time. Health workers do not know what to say or do for a patient that experiences chronic pain that does not respond to treatment. The person also has a tendency to talk about pain constantly. The nurse may believe that if he would only talk about something else, he would do better. However, you must remember that the pain is with this person constantly, so it is a major part of his life.

In providing care, communication is the single most important factor. The patient with chronic pain questions how he can be experiencing this. Convey your acceptance and belief to the patient regarding the presence of his pain by a willingness to listen carefully to what he says and to provide comfort measures that are indicated. Allow the patient to describe his pain, express his fears, anger, and frustration, and acknowledge the difficulty of the situation.

Involve the patient in discussion regarding pain and how to manage discomfort. Plan methods together to deal with the discomfort. In addition to pain medication, offer the patient pain-relief measures such as back rub, ice or heat application, relaxation techniques, and diversional activities. Encourage the patient to maintain an optimal activity level. To find out about the life of the patient, the nurse needs to talk with him. What can you do? What do you need assistance to do? How do you manage at home? What kinds of social activities are you able to do with your friends and families? What kinds of problems does your illness cause in your daily activities? Help the family of the patient to understand pain so they can cope and provide support to the individual with chronic pain. The patient with chronic pain is faced with multiple problems that require caring and support from his family and nurses.

◆ Homosexual Patient

Homosexuals are "coming out of the closet" in increasing numbers and are no longer carefully hidden.

Patients may tell you that they are homosexual. You should remember when caring for a homosexual patient that your responsibility is to the patient as a person who requires nursing care in a health care setting. Homosexual problems are more societal and have nothing to do with the nursing care you give.

As homophobia has increased, homosexual parents have difficulties obtaining custody of their children, adopting children, and getting married. If the patient wants to discuss problems of homosexual life, let the patient be the guide to how much and what is discussed. It is your responsibility to acknowledge homosexuality and discuss it freely, but remember privacy is a right of all patients.

◆ AIDS Patient

AIDS (acquired immunodeficiency syndrome) is an illness that is no longer associated only with homosexual or bisexual persons or intravenous drug users. It is a disease caused by the human immunodeficiency virus (HIV). Given the right circumstances, HIV can infect anyone, causing AIDS. As one report points out, for every child who meets the Centers for Disease Control definition for AIDS, 2 to 10 others may be infected with HIV.

AIDS carries a social stigma. Men especially fear being labeled as homosexuals should they develop AIDS. The parents of many AIDS babies do not want them, and the babies become wards of the state.

We all have personal views about AIDS. As nurses caring for patients with AIDS, we must examine our own feelings. In some cases the patient's family or friends may also be infected with HIV. Whatever the situation, it is important to be accepting and caring of the patient and his family and friends regardless of their situation.

If the nurse does not recognize life-styles that differ from the usual, then she will have difficulty caring for the AIDS patient and family.

It is the nurse's responsibility to ensure confidentiality for all patients, including the AIDS patient. Information should be given only to those health care professionals providing care for the individual. Information given to the wrong person about an AIDS patient could cause the patient to lose his job, home, and insurance. Some states have passed legislation to protect the privacy of AIDS patients.

Anger is frequently seen in AIDS patients. It may be directed at themselves for having taken a risk. If they have received a contaminated transfusion or because there is no cure available to them, anger may be directed toward the medical profession. The nurse needs emotional stamina but also needs to have a caring manner when the patient, family, or friends are showing their anger.

Because the patient inevitably will die, care of the AIDS patient is demanding. The nurse who begins to feel depressed, fatigued, or helpless should seek a support group and deal with her feelings openly. Some states are beginning to require AIDS education for nurses before licensure or relicensure to increase their knowledge in this area.

Because there is no cure at the present time, only symptomatic treatment is available for AIDS patients. Nursing care should take into consideration each patient's special needs and implement the care needed to meet them.

◆ Helping the Patient to Accept and Live With a Disease Condition

A patient cannot really accept his disease condition until he knows and understands it. This is his right. Just how much he is told and when he is told varies with the individual patient, his family, and his physician. The nurse who attempts to fulfill this function needs a good deal of psychological insight and understanding of the patient's personality to determine a wise course of action. It is certainly not desirable for you as a practical nurse to give this type of information. It is your responsibility to relate the patient's anxiety over the matter to your head nurse or team leader. Nevertheless, some things you can safely say to the patient. If a patient were to ask you, "Why are they doing this test?" you can safely answer him, sincerely and with concern, "These tests are being carried out so that the physician may find out definitely what is the matter with you." A simple explanation of the test may allay the patient's fears. In unknown situations the patient may be prone to build up imaginary horrors far worse than anything that is likely to happen. Never name the medications or types of dyes used in procedures because patients often tell their friends and relatives the name of a particular medication or tablet and may try to persuade them to take it also. Frequently they may have read an inaccurate report about the medication. As a result they may have distorted ideas about its effect on them and develop a fear of taking it.

It is the responsibility of the physician to determine how much information the patient is given. Sometimes the physician explains disease conditions in such a way that the patient is confused. Later the patient may ask the nurse to explain again what the doctor was trying to tell him. The nurse should know what the physician has told the patient before entering into a full explanation of the disease condition. The best way to gain this information is from the physician. In some cases the nurse may ask the patient to explain what he thought the physician was saying. If medical terminology was the stumbling block for the patient, a simple explanation may prove helpful. A rule to follow is "Never explain anything to a patient unless you know what you are trying to explain." Never bluff your way through an explanation. It is unfair to the patient and to your profession. Misinformation is harmful.

After the patient is informed and understands his disease condition, the nurse assists the patient in rehabilitation by use of a positive approach. It is easier to accept something positive rather than something negative.

The patient suffering from a crippling disease often can lead a productive life. With the aid of physical therapy and artificial devices, he may be taught to care for his own needs and pursue various occupations and recreational activities. Before this goal can be achieved, the patient must develop a desire to set such a goal. You can be of assistance to him in this area. Because you work so closely with him, ministering to his different needs, you can often give him the confidence he needs. Your trust in the patient is often sufficient to create this desire in him.

If the patient is completely helpless and still has full mental capabilities, he can be taught to use his mind rather than his hands or legs. He can further his education and find joy and happiness by reading, watching television, and listening to music. He can remain the head of the house, if this was his former position, by assuming and planning the household activities and finances. This takes a great deal of adjustment, but it can be done.

If he is not mentally alert, the patient may live in his own little world. He is happy because he is not cognizant of his former activities or of the world about him. He may find pleasure in making up fictional stories in which he is the main character. He is oblivious of all around him.

Is there a positive side to cancer? In some cases the patient dies as the result of the disease process; it may take weeks, months, or even years. Can you be sure that you will not die today or tomorrow? Death is as uncertain for you as for the patient with cancer. He may have many happy days to enjoy with his family. If he learns to live day by day, he may enjoy much happiness. Many new drugs and radiation therapy destroy cancerous cells and slow their growth.

If the patient's condition is terminal, he needs psychological, physical, and religious support. Encourage him to talk with his clergyman. However, he should not be forced into this. Listen to him. At such times of crisis the patient often looks for a sympathetic, understanding listener. Sometimes you are the one who can bring him the solace he is seeking. Your understanding may supply him with the courage he needs to face death bravely and peacefully. Death may be the blessing that ends his continuous suffering. By having his physical needs attended to with kindness and empathy, some of his psychological needs for love, affection, and acceptance are met. Many times it is more difficult to help the family to accept the situation than to help the patient.

◆ Dealing With the Patient's Family and Friends

Relatives and friends are important not only to the patient but also to the nursing staff. The patient is often lonely and longingly waits for his family. The nurse can gain real insight into the patient's needs by talking with relatives and friends. Many emotional, physical, and environmental factors are discovered through these interactions. The family may help the nurse to decide on the appropriate approach to use for this particular patient.

If you can establish favorable relations with relatives and friends, they are likely to be cooperative and helpful. It is true that the patient's relatives and friends at times present problems to the nursing staff in its daily routine. Some people exempt themselves from rules and visiting hours. They drop in to see the patient whenever it is convenient for them. They forget that certain functions or duties for the patient's comfort have priority. They may resent being told that they may visit only during the prescribed visiting hours. If you explain in a nonassuming, quiet voice these rules of the hospital and their purpose, often these persons are more willing to conform to them. If they persist, this should be reported to the head nurse, who will handle the situation.

When it becomes necessary to perform a procedure during visiting hours, ask the family or friends to kindly wait in the corridor or the waiting room for a few minutes. You may add that this procedure cannot wait until later. If you show them kindness, consideration, and respect, they will be willing to cooperate with anything that is of benefit to the patient. Remember that the patient, his family, and friends are guests in the hospital and should be treated as such.

Because of the crippling or finality of some disease conditions, families sometimes do not readily accept the sickness or misfortune inflicted on one of their loved ones. They tend either to reject it as nonexistent or to rebel against it. This rebellion may be against God, the medical profession, or society. The same procedure that is used to help the patient may be used to help the family. The family must know and thoroughly understand the disease condition and its implications, effects, and limitations. They must be helped to accept the condition before they can be of assistance to the diseased patient. Arrangements for the family to talk with the physician should be made at your earliest convenience. The help of the social service department may be sought to plan and contact various agencies that render the assistance needed. The family must be given understanding, guidance, and support. However, they must make their own decisions. The patient needs the family's help and depends on them. He senses and reacts to their reactions to his illness. Sometimes their clergyman may be of assistance. A positive approach to the patient and his family must be used to be effective. All must cooperate in the process of adjustment no matter which type of illness is involved. The degree of adjustment may necessarily differ, but it must be made. Its success depends on the persons involved and their acceptance of the illness.

For Study Helps, see next page.

◆ *Study Helps*

1. What determines the way you meet the special needs of your patients?
2. What is death?
   • List and explain the five stages of death.
   • State and explain an individual's concept of death as he matures.
   • Why are accidental deaths so difficult to understand?
   • How does religion affect the acceptance of death?
   • What can you do to assist a dying patient?
   • State and explain the family's reaction to death.
   • How can you be of assistance to the family?
3. Which complex needs do the elderly present?
   • What are their needs?
   • Where can they receive help?
   • What should be your attitude toward them?
   • What adjustments must they make?
4. Define and explain what is meant by the term *hostile, aggressive patient.*
   • Explain what is the most threatening and difficult situation for you as a practical nurse.
   • How should you cope with the situation?
   • What is meant by molestation?
   • Explain why the nurse is not guilty of molestation.
   • How does the belligerent patient differ from the hostile, aggressive patient?
5. What are the needs of the AIDS patient?
   • What are his reactions to illness?
   • How can you be of assistance to him?
6. What is the first step in helping a patient or his family to accept his illness?
   • What information can you as a practical nurse give to the patient or his family?
   • Which measures can be used to assist an invalid patient to adjust to his illness?
   • What assistance can you give to the seriously ill patient?
7. Explain the role of relatives and friends in the hospitalization of a patient.
   • How can you gain their cooperation?
   • How can you be of assistance to them in times of stress or crisis?
8. List three changes that take place in an aging person's life.
9. In which year was the abortion law liberalized?
10. What is your responsibility when you suspect child abuse?
11. List three characteristic behaviors that an alcoholic patient may display.

Bibliography

Barrick B: Caring for AIDS patients, *Nursing 88* 18:50-59, Nov 11, 1988.
Carpenito LJ: *Nursing diagnosis,* ed 4, Philadelphia, 1992, Lippincott.
Edelman CL, Mandle CL: *Health promotion throughout the life span,* ed 2, St Louis, 1990, Mosby.
Estes NJ, Heinemann ME: *Alcoholism,* ed 3, St Louis, 1986, Mosby.

Falco SA, McCormack AS: Intravenous therapy: attitudes of nurses and implications for managers and educators, *Geriatr Nurs* 12(4):207-209, 1992.

Gress LD, Bahr RT: *The aging person: a holistic perspective,* St Louis, 1984, Mosby.

Hamilton PM: *Basic pediatric nursing,* ed 6, St Louis, 1991, Mosby.

Kinney JK, Leaton G: *Loosening the grip: a handbook of alcohol information,* ed 4, St Louis, 1991, Mosby.

Kubler-Ross E: *On death and dying,* ed 4, New York, 1971, Macmillan.

Kubler-Ross E: *Living with dying,* New York, 1981, Macmillan.

Nick S: Long-term care—choices for geriatric residents, *J Gerontol Nurs* 18(7):11-18, 1992.

Potter PA, Perry AG: *Fundamentals of nursing,* ed 2, St Louis, 1990, Mosby.

Rogers FF: *Geriatric nursing care plans,* St Louis, 1991, Mosby.

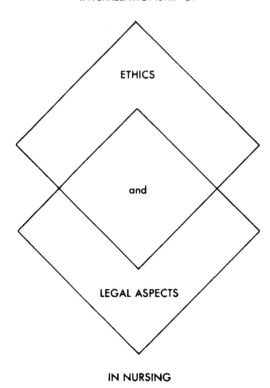

INTERRELATIONSHIP OF

ETHICS

and

LEGAL ASPECTS

IN NURSING

Influencing factors in nursing.

Objectives

At the completion of this chapter, the student practical nurse will be able to:

◆ Define the practice of nursing as a practical nurse.

◆ Discuss the terms *confidentiality* and *abandonment.*

◆ Describe the legal duty the nurse owes to a patient.

◆ Explain the purpose of the medical record.

◆ State why the study of ethics is important for nurses.

◆ Discuss ways a nurse can avoid a lawsuit.

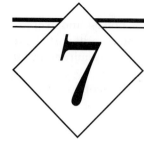

Legal and Ethical Issues in Practical Nursing

Mary Ann Shea

◆ Lawsuits—What Are They and Why Are There So Many?

What Is a Lawsuit?

A lawsuit is the result of legal action taken by a person or persons against another person or persons. The purpose is to make right some actual or perceived wrongdoing.

The person filing a medical malpractice lawsuit against a health care provider is called the *plaintiff* (also sometimes referred to as the *petitioner* or *claimant*). The person accused of the wrongdoing that allegedly injured the plaintiff is called the *defendant* (also sometimes referred to as the *respondent*). For purposes of this section we use the terms *plaintiff* and *defendant* to describe the parties to a lawsuit.

Lawsuits are being filed in record numbers. Often these lawsuits allege medical malpractice against a health care provider. Whereas physicians traditionally carried the brunt of malpractice risk, more and more nurses are now being named individually as defendants in medical malpractice lawsuits.

Lawsuits against nurses usually allege that the nurse failed to exercise the appropriate level of skill and training of a "reasonably prudent nurse." Another way to state this is that the nurse failed to abide by the appropriate nursing standard of care.

All health care providers are held to certain standards of care. The standards of care are different for the physician than for the registered nurse. Likewise, the standards of care for the registered nurse are different from those for the licensed practical nurse. It is imperative that nurses be aware of the applicable standards of care to which they will be held. Standards of care are derived from several sources, some of which are listed in the following discussion.

State licensing laws dictate certain parameters for nursing practice and requirements for licensure. All nurses by virtue of their licensure are expected to possess and exercise a certain level of skill and training. In addition, it is assumed that nurses will participate in continuing education, even though most states do not have such a requirement for relicensure. All nurses must keep their skills current.

Nurse practice acts, which exist in most states, broadly define the scope of nursing practice within that state. Nurses must be familiar with the provisions of their state's nurse practice acts.

Nursing organizations and associations exist for many specialty areas of nursing. Often these organizations and associations undertake the task of promulgating standards of practice. Each nurse must be familiar with these standards because it is assumed that each nurse is aware of them.

Journal articles often address current issues in nursing care and give recommendations as to how to deal with them. It is assumed that all nurses will maintain their skills according to current standards. For example, if an issue has been addressed in the *Journal of Practical Nursing,* the licensed practical nurse has a difficult time in court justifying why he or she was not aware of the current status of the issue.

Internal policies and procedures are generally written by the institution in which the nurse is employed. These are often quite specific. The nurse is expected to be familiar with *all* applicable policies and procedures of the employing institution and to abide by them faithfully.

Standards of care are used to determine what a nurse should or should not do. They can be used to prosecute or defend the nurse in determining whether the nurse lived up to the appropriate standard of care.

Why Are Lawsuits Increasing?

That the number of lawsuits is steadily increasing is not disputed. There are many reasons for this increase, some of which we explore in this chapter. The nurse must be cognizant of what motivates persons to file lawsuits if their goal is to minimize their chances of being sued. The best defense to a lawsuit is to *prevent* its being filed.

Litigious attitude. Our society is too willing to allow the courts to handle disputes. Problems that were formerly dealt with in a face-to-face confrontation now find their way to the courts. This is neither the most efficient nor the most cost-effective means of resolving disputes. Lawsuits cost all of us time and money.

Patient's expectations. The patient expects more from health care today than in the past. He also expects more from the nurse because the scope of nursing practice is continuously expanding. Formerly, only doctors were victims of lawsuits, but this has changed. The patient is now holding nurses accountable for their own independent actions.

Service. Our society is more service-oriented now than ever before, and the expectation of a high level of service now includes the health care profession. Patients seem intolerant of anything but the best level of service in meeting their needs. One of the most frequent patient complaints involves the *time* it takes to get what is needed, whether it is pain medication, a box of tissues, a bed pan, or just an answer to a call light.

Information and honesty. The patient expects the highest quality of care at all times. We are dealing today with persons who are well informed and are not timid about asking questions, often of the nurse instead of the physician. The patient expects honest answers. Consequently, the patient today is much more aware of when an adverse outcome occurs. Persons in our society also expect that "wrongs" will be compensated. So when something is wrong with his medical care, the patient is likely to pursue the legal remedies available to him.

Respect and privacy. The patient also expects to be treated with respect. He expects his privacy to be protected and expects to be treated with dignity at all times. For example, nurses are rather unaffected by the revealing nature of hospital gowns, but nurses must remember that the patient is often quite embarrassed by this exposure. Nurses must be sensitive to the patient's feelings about privacy.

Warm and caring nurse. The patient expects the nurse to display a warm and caring demeanor at all times. Despite the increasing complexity of nursing care and the evolution of the status as professionals, nurses are still perceived by patients as the kind and compassionate members of the health care team—the ones who hold the patient's hands and fluff their pillows. Unfortunately, when nurses are rushed by the everyday demands of modern nursing, patients might perceive them as cold and uncaring. This is a dangerous situation for the nurse from a liability perspective.

Every nurse knows that the time spent monitoring complex biomedical equipment benefits the patient and leads to immediate awareness of any changes in the patient's condition. But the patient's perception of this situation is different. When less time is spent on actual hands-on nursing care, the patient all too often perceives this as a *lack* of care.

The nurse must never underestimate the significance of the *patient's perceptions.* After all, it is often *not* what *actually* happens, but what the patient *perceives* happens, that leads to a lawsuit.

For example, a nurse enters a patient's room and obtains critical data regarding the patient's blood pressure, pulse, heart rhythm, respiratory status, oxygenation level, intake, and output—all without touching or talking to the patient. Then another nurse enters the same patient's room, talks to the patient, and takes hold of the patient's arm to take a blood pressure reading with a sphygmomanometer and stethoscope.

The patient's *perception* of the quality of nursing care given by the two nurses differs. The patient is more likely to feel "taken care of" by the second nurse, although the first nurse actually performed a more thorough and better quality assessment of the patient's condition. It is the patient's perception of the quality of care that reduces the likelihood of lawsuit against the second nurse.

◆ Common Bases for Lawsuits Against Nurses

Scope of Practice Issues

The licensed practical nurse must practice within the confines of the scope of practical nursing. Yet the reality of the current status of nursing is that there is a shortage of registered nurses. Because of this, the role of the licensed practical nurse has expanded over the years to include more responsibility for patient care and sometimes patient care management, a role formerly designated only to registered nurses. Whenever a nurse is faced with a trend toward expansion of practice, the nurse *must* be cognizant of the practice limitations imposed by law. Just because a patient has a need, the licensed practical nurse cannot necessarily fulfill the need within legal guidelines, if doing so requires that the licensed practical nurse operate outside the scope of practical nursing licensure restrictions. The prudent licensed practical nurse knows the limits of practice and operates within them at all times.

Autonomy

Another evolving trend in nursing that accompanies the general expanded scope of practice is that of autonomy. As nurses practice with more autonomy and independence, they automatically increase their risk of making errors for which they will be held accountable.

Practical nurses operate now with more autonomy than in the past. As practical nurses take on more charge type of responsibilities, the risk of making errors in judgment increases, as does the risk of being named as a defendant in a lawsuit.

This is not to say that autonomy is bad. On the contrary, it is a positive step in recognizing and appreciating the nurse's capabilities. But autonomy does lead to legal accountability for the nurse's actions.

Assessment and Reporting

Inherent in every nurse's role is the ability to properly assess a patient. Assessment is a basic function of nursing. A licensed practical nurse who does not understand the significance of a blood pressure of 60/40, cyanosis, or severe respiratory distress has no excuse for failing to recognize these abnormalities in a patient's condition. An allegation in a lawsuit of "failure to properly assess" a patient is difficult if not impossible to defend in court.

If the assessment of a patient reveals an abnormality, the nurse's obligation does not end. The nurse also has an obligation to intervene on the patient's behalf. The nurse must *report* the findings to the appropriate member of the health care team, such as the charge nurse, head nurse, or physician. Like failure to properly assess, failure to *report* abnormal findings of an assessment is also difficult to defend in court.

Falls

Many lawsuits are filed by patients who fall, but not all allege medical malpractice. Lawsuits involving falls generally come under two categories: those claiming general negligence and those alleging medical malpractice. Differentiating between the two requires an understanding of what it takes to prove medical malpractice against a health care professional.

To prove medical malpractice the plaintiff must establish by a preponderance of the evidence that four elements exist: the *duty* to the patient, the *breach* of the duty, an *injury* to the patient, and *causation* between the breach of the duty and the injury. If the plaintiff cannot prove all four elements, the plaintiff cannot prevail in court.

If a patient who is ambulatory and requires no assistance sustains an injury when he slips and falls in the shower of his hospital room, he might file a lawsuit. If he bases his lawsuit on the theory of medical malpractice against a health care professional, such as the nurse, he is not likely to be successful. This case is defensible by showing that a nurse generally has no *duty* to assist a patient who does not need assistance. One of the elements is missing, so the plaintiff has no case.

If an unsafe condition exists in the shower, such as a water leak onto the dry floor, an unsuspecting patient might slip and fall on the wet spot. If this patient sues, he might be successful in recovering for his injuries. This lawsuit, however, would not be filed against the nurse for medical malpractice but most likely against the hospital on a general negligence theory.

What if the nurse is caring for a patient who is unsteady and weak, and the nurse allows this patient to shower unassisted? If this patient falls and injures himself, is the nurse liable for the injuries? Yes, the nurse is liable for medical malpractice, because in this case the accident was related to a health care issue. The nurse in this case had a *duty* to assist a weak and unsteady patient in the shower, and the nurse *breached* the duty to the patient by failing to assist the patient. In addition, the *injuries* from the fall were *caused* by the breach of the duty.

The licensed practical nurse is often the team member most directly involved in hands-on patient care. Therefore the practical nurse must be aware of the high incidence of patient falls and the potential legal consequences for the nurse and the hospital when a patient fall leads to injuries and a lawsuit. Although many patients fall while in the hospital, fortunately not every patient fall results in a lawsuit, and of those that do, not all result in charges of medical malpractice against the nurse.

Medications

As more licensed practical nurses undertake the administration of medications, the number of lawsuits against them will undoubtedly increase. Many lawsuits result from problems involving medication administration. When you examine the amount of time the nurse spends in medication functions, it is not surprising that a large number of lawsuits involve medication issues. Some common medication errors are discussed next.

Wrong patient. Sometimes medication is given to the *wrong patient*. The nurse must realize that this action is seldom defensible in court, because the jury is not sympathetic to a nurse who fails to perform a simple procedure such as checking a patient's identification before giving medication.

Wrong medication. Sometimes the *wrong medication* is given to a patient. This is also difficult to defend in court. The nurse should always verify that he or she has the correct medication before administering it to a patient.

Wrong dosage. Giving the *wrong dosage* is another error. The nurse must be especially careful when decimal points are present. If 1.5 mg is ordered, receiving 15 mg might be detrimental to the patient.

Wrong route. Occasionally medications are given by the *wrong route*. The nurse cannot assume that a drug is to be given by the most common route. He or she must be certain that the route is clearly designated. Giving a dosage intramuscularly when it was meant to be given by mouth may result in an overdose.

Improper technique. Another issue involves *improper technique* used to administer medications. When giving intramuscular injections, it is imperative that the nurse use proper technique to avoid injuring the patient. Many lawsuits have been filed by patients who have sustained sciatic nerve injuries as a result of injections given in the wrong site. Careful site location techniques are essential to preventing this type of injury to a patient and thereby also preventing lawsuits.

Confidentiality

For health care to be of maximum benefit to the patient, the patient must often disclose to the health care team information of a very private and personal nature. To feel comfortable enough to make the necessary disclosures to the health care team, the patient must be able to trust that information conveyed in such a manner remains confidential. Without the assurance of confidentiality, information important to the treatment of the patient might not be given.

Patient information should only be available to those members of the health care team who are directly involved in the care of that patient. The nurse is usually the "watchdog" of the confidential information in the patient's medical record while the patient is hospitalized. Information about a patient should never be disclosed without the patient's authorization.

Consent

Proper informed consent must be obtained from the patient before treatment. Treating a patient without the patient's consent may result in a charge of *assault* or *battery*. Battery is the unauthorized touching of a patient, whereas assault is the threat of unauthorized touching. The defense to a charge of assault or battery is *consent*.

Nurses are often confused regarding their role in obtaining patient consent and the signing of consent forms. It is the physician's obligation to obtain informed consent from the patient. The consent form is *not* the same as the consent itself—it is a document for the medical record that verifies in writing that informed consent has been obtained. Informed consent is actually obtained during discussions between the physician and the patient about the proposed treatment, the risks, the expected outcome, and alternatives to the proposed treatment. The informed consent process often takes place in the physician's office before the patient is hospitalized.

Generally speaking, the nurse should not undertake the responsibility of obtaining informed consent. The nurse should approach the patient with the consent form and ask the patient if the physician has explained the procedures and answered all of the patient's questions. If the patient indicates that this has been done, the nurse should then ask the patient to read and sign the consent form. The nurse who witnesses the patient's signature is attesting that the patient stated that the physician had explained the procedure and answered all of his questions.

If a patient indicates that the physician has not explained the proposed treatment or if he has technical questions about the treatment, the nurse should *not* ask the patient to sign the consent form at that time. The nurse should relay to the physician that the patient does not understand the procedure or has questions about it. Only when the patient indicates that proper informed consent has been given should the nurse present the consent form to the patient for signing.

Abandonment

Several actions of a nurse can be categorized as abandonment. Leaving a unit unattended or understaffed, such as when a nurse leaves before the nurse's end-of-shift replacement arrives, may lead to a lawsuit based on abandonment if a patient suffers an injury because of the resulting shortage of staff. Likewise, if a nurse who is "pulled" to an unfamiliar unit refuses to go, and instead leaves rather than accepting the reassignment, that nurse could be sued for abandonment if a patient suffers harm because of the resulting inadequate staffing.

A charge of abandonment may also arise when a nurse fails to adequately observe or monitor a patient. If a nurse leaves a patient unattended for an inappropriate amount of time or fails to give care as directed, the patient may file a lawsuit if he is injured while not being attended by the nurse.

◆ Documentation

Even before your fingers cease contact with the previous page and as your eyes glance at the "Documentation" topic heading, you might feel an almost overwhelming temptation to simply skip this section and proceed to a less "undesirable" topic.

An amazing number of nurses feel this way. What is it about this all-important topic that causes the nurse to resist attempts to encourage compliance with documentation requirements?

To answer that question, nurses must first confront the fact that they generally tend to be "people-oriented." By nature they are the care-givers from whom others are supposed to benefit. Nurses are also the patients' advocate, constantly aware of their patients' welfare and protecting their patients from any compromises in effective care.

Nurses are *not* "paper-oriented" individuals. In fact, they view the paperwork aspect of their job as interfering with their real purpose, their real mission—patient care. Consequently, it is almost impossible for a nurse to recognize that both aspects—the care and the documentation—have significant consequences that, although quite different in purpose, are of similar importance.

This mind-set has created problems for the nursing profession. Nurses feel they are neglecting their patients when they take time out of their day—time they feel should be spent in hands-on nursing care—to document in the medical record. The nurse must realize that time spent documenting does not result in an abandonment of duty to the patient. On the contrary, *not* taking the necessary time to provide a medical record is the more frequent abandonment of duty of a licensed practical nurse.

How can this be? The evolution of nursing from "handmaiden" to "professional" status brought changes in the nurse's responsibilities. Without documentation a nurse is actually meeting only part of the responsibilities to the patient.

Based on the groundwork just laid, the next step is to discuss documentation in the necessary detail. This section addresses the purposes served by the medical record, documentation principles, common documentation problems to avoid, and what to expect if the nurse must go to court without good documentation.

Medical Record Purposes

The major purposes of a medical record may be divided into three categories. The primary purpose of the medical record is to provide for continuity of care. Second, it provides the basis for other hospital activities such as reimbursement, licensing, and accreditation. Third, it is a legal document that may be used to prove in court that the nurse provided the appropriate care for the patient.

Continuity of care. Providing for continuity of care is clearly the most important purpose for the existence of the medical record. The current practice of medicine involves a multidisciplinary approach to health care. Every patient has at least one, and sometimes several, physicians. Because health care is a 24-hour-per-day process, several shifts of nurses are involved in each patient's care. On each shift every patient might have several nurses and nurse assistants. In addition, other departments (such as physical therapy, respiratory therapy, laboratory, radiology, pharmacy, social service, pastoral care, and IV therapy) might be involved in administering care to a patient.

It is imperative that personnel in all ancillary services be aware of pertinent information about the patient. Information from all the different departments in a health care setting must be readily accessible to all members of the health care team. The medical record may be seen as the data bank from which all members of the health care team retrieve and input necessary information. Continuity of care cannot be achieved without a complete, accurate, and up-to-date medical record.

Although communication is the primary purpose of the medical record, it is not the only reason for its existence.

Other hospital activities. The medical record is a multipurpose document. The nurse is sometimes unaware of its significance in various ongoing hospital activities, such as in-hospital activities, reimbursement, licensure, and accreditation.

In-hospital activities. Documentation in the medical record forms the basis for many other in-hospital activities, such as utilization review, quality assurance, risk management, peer review, education, and research. Nurses often tend to view these activities as too remote from hands-on nursing care to be relevant to their daily practice, but this is not so. From these activities potential problems can be identified. The overall purpose of all these activities is identical to the goal of the majority of nurses—to provide the best and safest care possible for the patient.

Reimbursement. It may surprise some nurses, but documentation in the medical record often provides the basis for reimbursement decisions by third-party payers. Insurance companies often perform audits of medical records to determine whether they will assume financial responsibility for the treatment or hospitalization.

Sometimes insurance companies deny coverage because the medical record fails to substantiate the medical necessity for hospitalization or treatment. If the documentation in the medical record is incomplete or inadequate, the hospital might not be reimbursed for services it provides.

Licensure. All health care institutions must be licensed by the designated department in their state of operation. The state licensing department promulgates licensing requirements that the health care institution must meet to operate within that state. The licensing body of the state periodically performs in-depth audits of patient medical records to determine whether the quality of care meets its licensing requirements. If the documentation is inadequate, it is assumed that the care was also inadequate. It is easy to see how inadequate documentation leads to licensing problems for the institution. The consequences of losing state licensure are catastrophic for any health care institution.

As with the reimbursement issues discussed previously, good quality documentation that meets acceptable documentation criteria is also sufficient to ensure compliance with licensing standards.

Accreditation. Unlike licensing obligations, which are mandatory, accreditation is often sought voluntarily by health care institutions because most institutions recognize the necessity of accreditation.

The most well-known accreditation organization is the Joint Commission on the Accreditation of Healthcare Organizations (JCAHO). The JCAHO generally surveys each institution on a periodic basis. JCAHO standards on documentation must be met for the institution to be accredited. The nurse must be aware of the significance of quality documentation in this accreditation process. As with reimbursement and licensing, problems for the nurse arise only when the documentation is inadequate.

The nurse should never discount the importance of in-hospital activities, reimbursement, licensure, and accreditation, despite their perceived remoteness to the nurse's primary purpose of providing patient care. Nurses should also realize that by maintaining excellent documentation skills, the necessity of their involvement in these activities is minimized greatly, thereby freeing them to focus on their major concern—patient care.

Medical record as a legal document. In addition to its other purposes the medical record may also be used as a legal document. It is legally "discoverable" for purposes of legal investigation and litigation, which means it is admissible in court as evidence. Because of the manner in which medical records are recorded, and because they are completed close to the time of the event and before litigation is generally contemplated, they are presumed to be true and accurate.

The accuracy of the information in a medical record is difficult to refute. Because of this, the medical record is by far the nurse's *best* defense if the nurse is sued for medical malpractice.

Many types of cases, criminal and civil, reference the medical record in the pretrial investigations and court proceedings. These include the most obvious type of case—medical malpractice—as well as automobile accident cases, workers compensation, slip and fall cases, criminal assault, competency hearings, will contests, and child abuse and child custody cases. Actually, any cases in which a person's medical history might be an issue have the possibility of making their way into the legal system. And the nurse as the writer of the information might be called to testify.

Documentation Problems

We have previously addressed several purposes of the medical record. This section concentrates on the medical record from a *legal* perspective and explores some common documentation problems.

Inadequacies. The most common documentation problem is the *omission* of pertinent data. Incomplete charting tells only part of the story; it does not tell everything that was done for the patient. Nurses might believe that it is sufficient to "fill in the gaps" later with recalled events if a lawsuit is filed against them. Such naive practice is dangerous.

For a medical record to adequately defend the nurse in the event of a lawsuit, the record must clearly indicate that everything that was supposed to be done was in fact done—and done correctly. This is an awesome responsibility because it means that the medical record must tell the whole story, leaving nothing to the imagination of the jury. Unfortunately, an incomplete story allows listeners to fill in the gaps with whatever images come to mind, a practice that could be disastrous to the nurse.

If you are called to court to testify regarding treatment *not* documented in the medical record, the credibility of any facts "filled in" in the courtroom is at best questionable. Even though you are quite confident in your recollection of the events, both the documented events and those not documented, there is really no reason for the jury to believe your story instead of the plaintiff's story.

Jury perspective. To better understand the jury's perspective it is necessary to analyze the jury selection process. Before the trial the attorneys from both sides have the opportunity to interview, or "voir dire," each prospective juror. Then each attorney is allowed to "strike" certain jurors—to dismiss them. Attorneys obviously dismiss jurors with attitudes detrimental to their party's case. The goal is to select a group of jurors who have no preconceived ideas regarding who is right or who is wrong and who are willing to listen to all the evidence from both sides before determining who "wins."

We supposedly have a right to be judged at trial by a "jury of our peers." In reality this does not happen, because your peers are nurses, and the likelihood of any nurse being chosen to sit on the jury of a medical malpractice case is remote. The attorney for the plaintiff will strike that juror as being biased. But almost every juror has been a patient at some time. Consequently, the plaintiff is much more likely to be judged by a jury of peers. Unfortunately, the non-nurse juror is not capable of understanding how difficult it is to meet all documentation standards all the time, because the average juror has absolutely no idea what it is like to be a nurse.

The jury does know that two parties have conflicting stories and that both parties cannot possibly be telling the truth. Before the trial the jury does not know that you are a most kind and compassionate nurse who always gives the best quality care and that the plaintiff has distorted the facts to his benefit. The jury sees both parties on *equal ground*—neither more right than the other—at the onset of the trial. Even more frightening is the realization that the jurors are aware that the plaintiff and the nurse have a reason to lie!

With this basic assumption in place, reconsider the problems by trying to fill in the gaps of the medical record documentation with oral recounts of memories. Relying predominantly on the nurse's *spoken* words to support evidence in court is a dangerous practice, because the jury questions whether the spoken words are the truth, knowing that the nurse has a motive to not speak the truth! In addition, the plaintiff is filling in these same gaps with a completely different story.

Because both accounts of the events that took place are elicited during a trial, both accounts are considered by the jury to be self-serving and therefore not necessarily believable. This presumption puts both parties back on equal ground, a place you do not want to be. In front of a jury, having the competitive edge is the desired position. This edge is gained by presenting evidence considered credible by the jury. By far the most credible evidence in any lawsuit is the documentation in the medical record. If the record is complete and tells the whole story, the jury will believe the medical record.

Documentation Do's and Don'ts

A poorly written medical record is like a time bomb sitting quietly and without repercussion, giving the writer a false sense of complacency disproportionate to the danger that might lurk ahead.

The writer seldom receives immediate negative feedback for a poorly written record. The delayed repercussions of poor documentation make the problem more difficult to correct because many nurses have never experienced the negative results of poor documentation habits.

But it is likely that sooner or later the nurse will get caught off guard in court with an incomplete or poorly written medical record. Only then does the time bomb explode, inflicting significant wounds on the writer with the shrapnel of inadequate documentation. There are seldom any minor injuries, only deeply penetrating wounds resulting in permanent scarring.

Going to court is not fun. Going to court without a well-written medical record is like having surgery without anesthesia. It is a painful experience. Unfortunately, many nurses wait until it is too late before changing their documentation habits.

Going to court is probably the most effective method for teaching what should and should not be documented in the medical record, but that is not to say it is the best way to learn. Those who have been involved in litigation can probably tell you that the experience changed the way they document. But there are better, less dramatic, ways to learn good documentation techniques.

So how can you improve your documentation skills? First, you must recognize your charting inadequacies, and then make the *commitment* to yourself to improve them.

Some common documentation issues are listed below with suggestions as to what to do and not to do.

Always document in ink. The nurse's documentation is part of the patient's permanent record. Entries done in pencil are *not* necessarily permanent and can be tampered with. The astute nurse does not let this happen. Always documenting in ink removes this risk.

Always write legibly. Unreadable documentation cannot communicate information. In the event of a lawsuit the nurse may be called on to "translate" an unreadable note for the jury. The nurse will hopefully be able to do so. If the nurse cannot, it is synonymous with not having provided any documentation and therefore not having provided the care. Remember, if it wasn't charted, it wasn't done! An unreadable note cannot help the nurse win a lawsuit.

Always include the date and time on all entries. Nursing documentation is an ongoing process. The more specific the time of the entries, the more the entry protects the nurse in the event of a legal challenge. Nurses should generally avoid long time spans for block charting, such as an entry timed 7 AM to 3 PM. This type of entry creates problems for the nurse in defending a lawsuit, because something that occurred during the shift may be of no legal significance if it happened at 2:45 PM but may be of tremendous legal significance if it happened at 7:15 AM. If the medical record clearly states that the time of occurrence was 2:45 PM, such an entry defends the nurse in court. One that simply states something happened sometime between 7 AM and 3 PM does not.

Always document omitted information as a "late note." A late note is better than no note at all. Nurses are human and do sometimes forget to write things down at the time they are performed. To ensure the credibility of a late note, it must be clear from reading the entry that it has been written out of sequence. Do not try to hide this fact. Whenever the nurse realizes that pertinent information has been omitted from a patient's chart, a late note should be written. Obviously, the best defense is provided when the late note is documented as close to the time of the occurrence as possible. A note added 3 hours late has much more credibility than one entered a month later.

Never obliterate an entry in a medical record. Obliterations may be used by the opposing attorney to imply a cover-up. Never use opaquing liquid or anything else to completely cover any documentation. Always follow your institution's policy for correcting documentation errors.

Nurses should draw a single line through the incorrect entry, making sure it can still be read. Keep in mind that an obliterated note may easily be used by the opposing attorney to fill in the obliteration with whatever statement benefits the plaintiff. Unfortunately, the nurse might not be able to defend the allegation because the nurse cannot prove the true content of an obliterated note.

Never leave blank lines in the medical record. Most nurses have at one time or another been asked to save a "couple of lines" for someone else to document something in the medical record at a later time. The requester often discovers later that the added documentation did not fit in the requested space. The result is a record that obviously was *not* completed in chronologic order. This improper procedure is sure to be confronted by the plaintiff's attorney who may use it to discredit the credibility of the entry and those surrounding it.

Never use the patient's medical record to air disputes. Never use the chart to criticize the actions of other members of the health care team. Other, more appropriate formats are available to air disputes with doctors or other team members. The patient's medical record should contain only information pertinent to the patient's care. When documenting information for which a conflict exists, remember to be objective at all times. Avoid making judgmental comments in the medical record.

Always document objectively. *Objective* data reflects what we hear, see, feel, or smell. *Subjective* information is often opinion. Objective data accurately conveys what happened. Subjective data, opinions, and judgmental comments do not. Subjective comments are open to several interpretations. Objective comments are not. For example, documenting that a patient is "disoriented" is subjective and may be interpreted several ways. Stating that a patient "does not know his name, where he is, or what day it is" is objective and conveys specific information. Use your senses to obtain the data for your documentation.

Always document patient's noncompliant behavior. Often the nurse is well aware of a patient's noncompliance with recommended treatment. This information should be documented objectively in the patient's medical record. The bulemic patient who is observed binging and the diabetic patient who refuses to follow dietary restrictions are contributing to their own demise despite conscientious medical care.

If a noncompliant patient brings a lawsuit, the jury has a right to know about these self-destructive behaviors. The defense of comparative fault or contributory negligence can then be raised in court. The doctor or nurse should not be held accountable for problems the patient caused.

◆ Ethical Issues

Conflicts in health care are not limited to legal issues. Ethical dilemmas also lead to conflicts for the nurse.

Ethical dilemmas are difficult for the nurse because there is seldom clear direction as to which approach is right and which is wrong. The problem is that equally strong moral values drive those on *both* sides of ethical controversies.

The patient's right to refuse treatment and die with dignity and the nurse's refusal to participate in treating select patient groups, such as those who have acquired immunodeficiency syndrome (AIDS) or those undergoing abortions, are just a few of the ethical concerns in health care today.

Right to Refuse Treatment and Die with Dignity

The right to refuse treatment and the right to die raise many medical, legal, and ethical questions as modern technology provides the capability of elaborate life-support systems. Most health care professionals recognize that just because we have the capability to sustain "life" indefinitely, we should not always do so.

The patient has a right to refuse unwanted treatment, as long as the patient is a competent adult (on whom no minor children depend solely for support). The problem arises when a patient is incapable at the time of making or communicating the decision to refuse treatment. The courts have dealt with these issues for years, trying to balance the wishes of the families to refuse treatment on behalf of the patient against the government's interest in preserving life. Consequently, it is sometimes difficult to convince a court to allow the substituted judgment of the family to make a decision that will ultimately end the life of another person.

It is widely accepted that the patient has the right to determine what medical treatment he will accept or refuse. The patient is setting out *prospectively* what treatment he wants and does not want in the event he *later* becomes unable to participate in the consent or refusal decisions. These documents come in many forms, the most common of which are living wills, advanced directives, durable powers of attorney for health care, and do-not-resuscitate (DNR) orders.

Living wills and *advanced directives* are more similar than different. They are patient-initiated documents that are drafted while a patient is mentally competent and that set out in varying detail what treatments the patient will accept or refuse in the event he later becomes mentally incapacitated. A *durable power of attorney for health care* is a document drafted by the patient that designates a proxy decision maker to consult in the event the patient cannot make his own treatment decisions. The person to whom the durable power of attorney for health care is granted then becomes responsible for making decisions regarding the patient's medical treatment and can consent to or refuse treatment on the patient's behalf.

The patient is not usually involved in the physician's decision to write a *DNR* order. A DNR order is usually the result of a decision made by the physician and the patient's close relative or relatives. It presumably reflects the patient's wishes as communicated by those closest to the patient.

The nurse is the patient advocate and as such must do whatever possible to assure that these documents are honored. Often a nurse is involved in the care of a patient who has clearly set out his wishes in a living will or advanced directive but who has a relative who pressures the health care team to do more than the patient wants. Unfortunately, some physicians bend to the pressure of the family, fearing reprisals from them, and treat the patient despite advanced directives not to do so. When confronted with such a situation, the nurse must intervene as *patient advocate* by notifying the appropriate personnel in the chain of command. This usually involves informing the charge nurse, head nurse, supervisor, or the medical director. The nurse must always remember that it is the *patient's* choice, not the family's, that is first.

Refusal to Treat

Sometimes nurses encounter situations that cause conflict with their own moral beliefs. It is important that the nurse know when he or she can and cannot refuse to render treatment to a particular patient.

Abortion is one of the most heated controversies existing today. If a nurse who believes that abortion is morally wrong is assigned to assist with an abortion, that nurse may communicate to the supervisor that he or she cannot morally or ethically participate in such a procedure. The nurse may also request reassignment, which should be granted. It is important that the nurse follow proper procedures in declining the abortion assignment—simply walking out and "abandoning" the patient may lead to serious repercussions.

On the contrary, the nurse *cannot* refuse to participate in the care of a person who has had an abortion just because the nurse does not agree with the patient's actions. Nurses cannot be judgmental in treating patients. From a nursing point of view, a criminal deserves the same standard of nursing care as the crime victim.

Likewise, the nurse has no legal right to refuse to care for a patient who has AIDS.

◆ Defenses—How to Avoid Lawsuits

Prevention is the best defense to a lawsuit. If the lawsuit cannot be prevented, a well-written medical record provides the second best defense. The nurse who wants to stay out of court should always remember the following three *D*'s of medical malpractice defense: dedication, demeanor, and documentation.

Dedication to competency is of primary importance in avoiding lawsuits. The licensed practical nurse must know and do what is expected by virtue of licensure and must always abide by the appropriate standard of care. The licensed practical nurse must maintain the highest level of competency at all times, including maintaining skills through continuing education. A dedicated nurse always gives the best quality care.

The nurse's *demeanor* is often the determining factor in whether the patient sues the nurse. A warm and caring demeanor may prevent a lawsuit. The nurse must never underestimate the significance of demeanor and rapport in malpractice prevention.

Documentation in the medical record provides the only credible proof in court that the appropriate care was given and the standard of care was met. Always remember that if it wasn't charted, it wasn't done.

The nurse who is conscientious about the three *D*'s of defense significantly minimizes the risk of ending up in court.

◆ *Study Helps*

1. Define the term *lawsuit*.
2. Why are lawsuits increasing?
3. List three patient expectations.
4. Name four common bases for lawsuits against nurses.
5. What is the importance of the patient's chart in legal action?
6. Give five do's and don'ts in patient documentation.
7. What ethical issues arise while caring for patients?
8. What are the major purposes of the medical record?

Bibliography

Carbary LJ: How to help prevent falls, *J Prac Nurs: 13-49,* June 1991.
Creighton H: *Law Every Nurse Should Know,* ed 5, Philadelphia, 1986, WB Saunders.
Fuetz-Harter SA: *Nursing and the Law,* ed 4, 1991, Professional Education Systems.
Hart PD: What the public thinks, *J Prac Nurs: 29,* March 1991.

Hollowell EE, Eldridge JE: Drug and alcohol abuse: medical record confidentiality, *J Prac Nurs: 46-49,* March 1989.

Hollowell EE, Eldridge JE: Elderly patients and mature decisions: the right to a natural death, *J Prac Nurs: 44-47,* September 1988.

Hollowell EE, Eldridge JE: The disclosure of patient care errors by nurses: what duty owed? *J Prac Nurs: 42-45,* September 1988.

Hollowell EE, Eldridge JE: The nurse's role in informed consent, *J Prac Nurs: 28-31,* September 1989.

Hollowell EE, Eldridge JE: The nursing shortage: the increased risk of legal liability and how to avoid it, *J Prac Nurs: 28-31,* June 1989.

Huerta SR, Oddi LF: Refusal to care for patients with human immunodeficiency virus/acquired immunodeficiency syndrome: issues and responses, *J Prof Nurs 8(4): 221-230,* 1992.

Kazanowski MK: A nursing department's response to risks associated with human immunodeficiency virus, *Nurs Outlook 40(1): 42-44,* 1992.

Kjervik DK: The choice to die, *J Prof Nurs 7(3): 151,* 1991.

Locher CJ: How to make the most of your charting, *J Prac Nurs: 35-43,* June 1992.

Merker L: Meet the challenge: health care in the 1990's, *J Prac Nurs: 32,* September 1991.

Miller I, Kjervik DK: The safe medical device act of 1990—ethical dilemmas for nurses, *J Prof Nurs 8(5): 260,* 1992,

Schwarz JK: Living wills and health care proxies: nurse practice implications, *Nurs Health Care, 13(2): 92-96,* 1992.

Self C: Practical problems that commonly arise in medical lawsuits, *J Prac Nurs: 48-49,* September 1992.

Weber G, Kjervik DK: The patient self-determination act—the nurse's proactive role, *J Prof Nurs 8(1): 6,* 1992.

Weiler K: Functional assessment in the determination of the need for a substitute decision maker, *J Prof Nurs 7(6): 328,* 1991.

Weiler K: Substitute decision makers in health care treatment decisions, *J Prof Nurs 7(5): 268,* 1991.

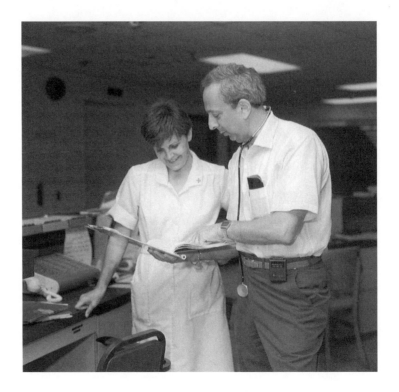

Objectives

At the end of this chapter the student practical nurse will be able to:

◆ Discuss the supervisory role of the practical nurse

◆ Explain basic principles of group dynamics

◆ Identify selected methods of dealing with conflict

◆ Explain the role of communication in supervision

◆ Identify ways of maintaining motivation in the workplace

◆ Describe the legal issues and guidelines related to delegation

◆ Discuss methods for dealing with problem employees

◆ Identify personal values as they relate to leadership

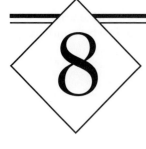

Leadership and the Practical Nurse

Gloria E. Wold

◆ Need for Leadership Skills

Because of today's nursing staff shortage in the United States, the health care delivery system requires that each person work to the maximum potential. With the shortage of nurses and the increasing demand for health care by society, the licensed practical nurse (LPN) is called on to perform many functions and accept multiple responsibilities. This is particularly true in long-term and extended care facilities. Although each state has different laws and agency policies, the practical nurse is increasingly likely to supervise other employees. Frequently she is expected to function as the charge nurse or team leader. She is expected to supervise aides and nursing assistants and to coordinate the day-to-day activities of a ward, unit, or wing.

Frequently an LPN is new to an institution when she is assigned "charge" responsibilities. Not only is she expected to perform skilled nursing care (observational changes, medications, and treatments) for a large number of patients, but also she is expected to supervise and coordinate the work of other less-skilled personnel. This is a great deal of responsibility to assume in a short period. These expectations are unreasonable, but unfortunately this occurs frequently. This amount of responsibility, assumed too quickly, often causes the practical nurse to become frustrated; feeling lost and frustrated, she tries to do the best she can. The training has not prepared her for the added responsibilities.

Because of limited time, many nursing schools focus on the clinical nursing skills. Leadership and supervision skills often are not addressed. This gap in nursing education is understandable; technical nursing knowledge has expanded so quickly that there is not enough time to teach everything. This is unfortunate, however, because without quality leadership and supervision, patient care suffers. Some students are fortunate;

111

they seem to be born leaders and adapt easily to the supervisory role. These are the fortunate few. Most students learn leadership skills over a period of time by trial and error. It is hoped that this material makes the transition easier for you.

◆ Legal Implications

Before you accept the responsibilities of team leader or charge nurse, you must be aware of the *allowable scope of practice* for a practical nurse in your state. In most states the practical nurse works under the direction of a registered nurse, physician, or other approved medical personnel. This scope is interpreted differently in each state, and sometimes even in different areas of the same state. No textbook can address all of the variations adequately. It is important that you discuss this topic in class so you have a clear understanding of the laws in your state. It is imperative that you do not exceed your legal limitations. Ignorance of the law does not protect you. When dealing with organizational or supervisory problems or situations in which complex judgments must be made, be sure to seek guidance from your manager. This is similar to what you have learned to do in patient care situations. When a nursing situation regarding a patient becomes too complex or exceeds your level of practice, notify the registered nurse or physician.

When you supervise others, the same principle is true. When a situation exceeds your scope of practice, you must seek guidance. You should not be expected to deal with these situations on your own.

◆ Attitudes, Beliefs, and Leadership

Before you attempt to lead or supervise others, knowing something about yourself is essential. Your values and beliefs determine to a large extent your attitudes and actions. Knowledge of your unique strengths and weaknesses enables you to develop a plan that develops and builds on your strengths and minimizes your weaknesses.

The nurse who is sincerely interested in others, who is a good listener, who tries to understand others and learn from them, and who enjoys working with others to achieve goals is most likely to be a successful leader and supervisor.

Values clarification exercises and a listening skills quiz at the end of this chapter may help you understand yourself better and determine the strengths and weaknesses you bring to the leadership role. This self-evaluation is a necessary starting point for anyone who hopes to lead others effectively.

◆ Management and Supervision

Management refers to the highest levels of the organization and is also used to describe the activity of directing the actions of a large number of persons. High-level managers or administrators are responsible for making an organization or business succeed. They have a great deal of authority and responsibility. The higher they are in the organizational structure, the greater their responsibility and authority. Some tasks involved in management include planning, preparation of budgets, hiring, firing, and supervising employees. In general, managers look at the "big picture" concerns of the institution.

Supervision involves directing and inspecting the day-to-day work performance of others. Supervisors usually are in the middle levels of the organization. They have various levels of authority, depending on the institution. Usually they work under the direction of a manager. Supervisors have the responsibility to see that selected tasks are completed either by themselves or by the people they supervise.

◆ Leadership and Supervision

Leadership and supervision are often defined as accomplishing tasks through others. No one person can do everything. Getting things done frequently requires a group effort. To be a good leader and supervisor it is important to understand more about groups and group dynamics.

Leadership Styles

Leadership styles are discussed in Appendix B. A self-test is provided in Appendix C to help you determine your preferred style of leadership. It may also help you determine your preferences when working with your supervisor.

Groups and Group Dynamics

A group is two or more persons who often have a common goal. Groups may be large or small, simple or complex, formal or informal. Some examples are businesses, hospitals, families, churches, work teams, clubs, or study groups. Large groups often have several smaller groups within them. Groups take on personalities of their own. Groups have values, and rules are established to guide the behavior of members.

Organizations such as businesses or hospitals have written goals because of their size and complexity. These are called the philosophy, mission statement, or strategic plan of the organization. Managers have developed a formal organizational structure to regulate and govern the organization. Fig. 8-1 shows how the individuals and groups within the organization relate to each other. In most situations a hierarchy is formed. This hierarchy illustrates how information moves. The figure also shows the flow of power or authority. The organization sets up rules that outline acceptable behaviors and also defines the rewards and punishments for appropriate and inappropriate behaviors. These rules are found in policy and procedure manuals.

Each person in a formal group is assigned a role. In an organization this becomes a job description, which includes a list of duties and responsibilities. Decisions and changes occur slowly in large organizations because a large number of persons are involved, and because fixed structures and rules resist change.

The structure and dynamics of smaller, less formal groups such as families, work groups, or friends who study together are not as easily described. Informal groups have unwritten goals and values. They accept or reject certain behaviors from their members. Each informal group is unique. The members know the rules in their own group. They know how information moves through the group and who the leader is, but an outsider is usually not aware of how each informal group works.

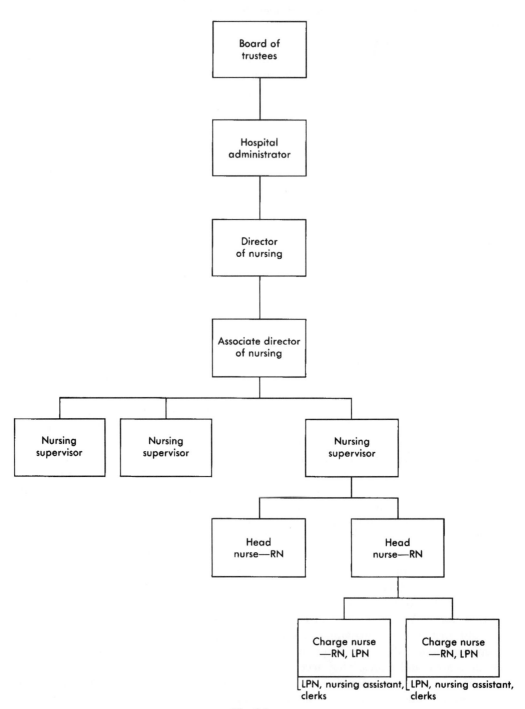

Fig. 8-1

Within informal groups the same person may have several different roles. Decisions and changes are made quickly to respond to the needs of the group. Good observation and communication skills are required if an outsider wants to determine the values, flow of information, and power structure of an informal group.

Conflict

Every person is a member of many different groups. Think for a moment. Try to identify all of the different groups to which you belong. There are groups at home, at school, at work, and in the community. Within one area such as work, each individual may belong to several different formal and informal groups. For example, one person may be a member of the LPN group, the charge nurse/supervisor group, the night shift, the 3-West team, and a member of the infection control committee.

When the goals and values of the formal and informal groups are in harmony and support each other, activities usually go smoothly. Large amounts of work can be accomplished, and people are happy and satisfied while doing the work.

Problems arise when the goals and values of two groups differ significantly, or when one group does not understand the viewpoint of another group. When there is a great deal of difference in values or goals between groups, misunderstandings and conflicts occur. These are manifested as anger, hostility, and resistance, which result in even less communication between the groups. The persons involved are unhappy and dissatisfied. Work performance and productivity levels are low. In a health care setting this affects the patients, who become the innocent victims.

Internal conflict and stress occur when a person has loyalty divided between several groups. If the groups have different goals and values, individuals feel that they are being pulled in different directions by each group. They are not sure which goals or values are right. They often try to please everyone and yet feel that they are not pleasing anyone. Frustration, guilt, and loss of effectiveness and sometimes even physical symptoms such as headaches result.

You can probably list many conflict situations from personal experience. Simply identifying problems does not help when you are the person in charge.

An individual may respond to conflict in different ways. The type of response depends on the importance of the outcome, the time available, and the persons involved. No one right way to resolve conflicts exists, but some methods are more effective than others. The approach that is right in one situation may be wrong in another. Conflict resolution is to a great degree situational. The following are some ways of dealing with conflict:

1. *Avoidance or "leaving well enough alone."* Avoiding conflict may occasionally be desirable. When the issues at conflict are either too minor or too great to resolve, when attempts to resolve the conflict may damage relationships or cause even greater problems, and when there is no chance of accomplishing a goal, it may be best to avoid the issues and leave the conflict well enough alone.
2. *Accommodation or "killing with kindness."* Accommodation is useful when being right is less important than the risk of damaging a relationship. It is useful when the issues at dispute are more important to the other person than to yourself and when you are willing to allow someone to learn from their mistakes.

3. *Authoritarian or "might makes right."* Use of authority is necessary when a decision is required in an emergency situation or when an unpopular decision must be made. It is also useful when dealing with a person who takes advantage of others. The authoritarian position resolves conflict by eliminating options.

4. *Compromise or "splitting the difference."* Compromise is effective when the outcome is moderately important but not worth excessive expenditure of energy. It also is useful when two individuals are equally committed to mutually exclusive goals or when a temporary resolution must be achieved in a complex problem.

5. *Collaboration or "two heads are better than one."* Collaboration is best when the outcome is too important to settle through compromise. It is useful when the objective is to increase understanding or insight into another's perspective or when feelings are interfering with interpersonal relationships.

◆ Communication Skills

Communication skills are essential to all phases of life. You have learned about communication from the first day you entered nursing school. An earlier chapter of this text gives a good review of some basic principles. The relationship of communication to supervision has been referred to as one and the same thing. An effective supervisor is an effective communicator. Review the following skills and apply them to supervision.

Listening

Listening to others is the most difficult communication skill to acquire. Many things get in the way of effective listening. Hearing is not listening. Listening requires close attention and concentration. Ineffective listening results in confusion, wasted time, and poor morale and is potentially harmful to patients. For example, while caring for a patient, you observe a change in vital signs. You report this to the team leader who is passing medications. You think it is important that she have this information promptly, because the physician is due in the unit shortly. She "listens" to you, but 15 minutes later when the physician arrives she calls you away from your duties to get the current vital signs for the same patient. Remember, it is easy to see this behavior in someone else, but difficult to see in ourselves. A short quiz on listening skills at the end of the chapter may give you an idea of how good a listener you are.

The following list identifies some common listening blocks to communication and offers more effective actions that the supervisor may take.

Listening blocks	Effective listening techniques
Too busy with something else	Focus on the message. If you are too busy, explain this and schedule a time when you can give your full attention. Write down information when it is given to you.
Too busy thinking about reply to listen	Focus on what the speaker is saying, not on what you are thinking.
Not interested in the message or pretends to listen	Recognize that as the supervisor you should be interested in your staff and all aspects of patient care.

| Too many distractions | Find a quiet place to talk away from the nurses' station and telephone. |
| Thinks she already knows what the message is | Verify the information. Ask questions until you are sure you have the correct facts. |

Although listening is a large part of communication, sending messages appropriately is also an important skill for the supervisor.

Verbal Communication

In supervision you are called on to give directions and information to your staff. You are the bridge between the policies of the formal organization and the day-to-day work. You must deliver messages, coordinate activities, and give specific information regarding the patients and the tasks that need to be done. The following are suggestions for improved verbal communication:

Make sure you have the other person's attention before speaking, particularly if you are giving directions.

Select a location for communication that is free from excessive noise or distractions.

Think and organize the message before speaking.

Use clear, concise, understandable language and avoid the use of highly technical terminology.

Watch your body language when delivering a verbal message.

Written Communication

At times a written message is more appropriate than a verbal one. Written messages are tangible. They may be referred to whenever needed. If you do not want instructions to be forgotten or missed, write them down.

As a supervisor you may be expected to communicate in writing to other departments in the facility. These are some times you want to be sure to put things in writing:

Any time a record of the message may be needed at a later time. For example, when making assignments, it is best to back them up in writing so there is no confusion about responsibilities.

When much of the material is new to the worker. New employees may require more written information on the assignment sheet.

If the message is complicated or has several steps.

When the message is sent to someone in another area or on another shift.

When the same message goes to several different persons.

When you do use the written method of communication, be sure that your thoughts are clearly written. Use correct grammar and punctuation, and make sure that your writing is legible.

Nonverbal Communication

You may talk about the need to give quality care and respond to patients promptly, but are you a good role model? If a signal light goes on, do you answer it, or do you excuse yourself because you are busy with something else? As the charge nurse you have many responsibilities that you cannot delegate to your assistants, but if they are busy and you have time, help them. Let your actions show cooperation and team spirit. Demonstrate the types of response and interaction you want them to have with patients. If you want to receive courteous treatment, then you must treat others, including your staff, courteously.

◆ Maintaining Motivation in the Workplace

Nursing is hard work. Few professions demand so much from a person for so few tangible rewards as does nursing. The nurse who provides for the day-to-day needs of patients usually does so for reasons other than financial gain. She often is motivated by a need to feel that she is needed, that what she does is important, and that she can make a positive difference in the lives of her patients. Often the care giver such as the nurse loses motivation. She often feels stressed and depressed when in spite of long, often exhausting hours she is unable to feel that she really is accomplishing anything. High levels of stress generally result in decreased effectiveness and a decline in the level of patient care, which in turn only increase the stress. If this cycle persists, the nurse and other care givers "burn out" and lose their motivation.

Stress may be manifested in many ways, such as increased level of frustration, loss of emotional control, increased frequency of arguments or other conflicts, increased use of alcohol or drugs, increased absenteeism, and increased stress-related illness. Dedicated nurses may even leave the profession.

The nurse, particularly one who supervises others, must take deliberate measures to reduce stress for herself and those with whom she works. Some measures that help reduce stress are as follows:

1. Set attainable work loads and standards. Remember you are not "Supernurse."
2. Ask for suggestions on how to improve the work climate and incorporate these suggestions when possible.
3. Compliment persons on what they did right. Don't be afraid to give praise to your employees when it is deserved. Give yourself positive affirmations to keep up your own self-esteem.
4. Celebrate small successes and find frequent reasons for celebration. Positive feelings are just as contagious as negative ones. Celebrations are an antidote to depression and stress.
5. Observe good health practices and encourage your staff to do likewise. Get enough rest, good food, and exercise. These all help you cope with stress.
6. Do the best job you can when you are working, but when you go home, leave the job behind.
7. Find something you enjoy doing and do it! Recharge your batteries away from work so you have the energy and motivation to face the stressors that are inevitable.

◆ Delegation

Supervision includes delegation, which is the assignment or entrusting of certain acts or duties to others. Nursing practice acts often include statements regarding delegation. "Delegated medical acts" are acts that are delegated to the registered nurse or LPN by the physician. "Delegated nursing acts" are those acts delegated to the LPN or less skilled assistant by the registered nurse. The LPN working as a charge nurse often delegates selected nursing activities to the nursing assistants.

Delegation is necessary because highly educated and skilled care givers are too few to meet the demands placed on the health care system. Delegation releases the most highly trained people to do the most important or most skilled work. Delegation extends the ability of an individual to achieve results. Results expand from the limited number of activities that one individual can do to the larger number of activities that the individual can control.

Caution must be used when work is delegated to others. Just as the LPN must be careful to accept assignments that are within her scope of practice, the LPN must be careful to delegate tasks appropriately. Tasks that *should not be delegated* include the following:

Tasks that are your specific responsibility

Tasks that other individuals are not adequately trained to perform

Tasks that you are not willing to do yourself

Tasks that *may be delegated* include the following:

Tasks that come within an individual's abilities and level of training

Tasks that help an individual grow and develop

Tasks that utilize an individual's unique talents

Delegation of tasks does not remove the nurse's responsibility. The nurse who delegates work to another less skilled individual remains responsible to see that any care delegated is performed safely and completely. All delegated work requires either direct or general supervision from the person who delegated the work.

Tact and concern for your assistants are an important part of delegation and supervision. Good relationships with those under your supervision may be facilitated by following certain guidelines, which are these:

1. All assistants should be treated respectfully and as adults. Assuming an "I'm better than you" attitude is counterproductive to the development and maintenance of positive working relationships. The nurse should be open and available to the assistants and should work to establish a climate in which assistants feel comfortable asking questions and seeking guidance.

2. The nurse should set definite expectations for work performance and communicate these clearly to the assistants. A specific time and place should be set aside for giving reports and directions so that full attention is devoted to the communication. The work assignments should be clearly described. Directions should be kept simple, brief, and concise with the focus on the information the assistants need to know. The nurse should be careful to avoid excessively technical terminology that assistants might not understand. Make sure that assistants are apprised of any changes in directions throughout the day. When changes are made, it is wise to ask assistants to repeat or restate the changes in directions to make sure that they clearly understand what is expected.

3. Be sure to allow adequate time for your assistants to question or clarify directions, particularly if these are in any way unusual or different from familiar routines. If directions are complex, they are best communicated in writing so that assistants have something to which to refer for clarification.

4. The nurse should continue to communicate with assistants throughout the day and give feedback regarding their progress. The nurse should be careful to observe their performance and should verify that all delegated tasks are performed safely and completely. If the nurse determines that an assistant's performance is not satisfactory, corrective actions should be taken promptly. This may involve teaching, additional explanations and clarification, or referral to higher levels of supervision if disciplinary action is required.

5. In addition, the nurse should verify that the assistants have all of the supplies or other resources needed to perform the delegated tasks. This includes making sure that all equipment is in proper working order. The nurse should do everything possible to facilitate the work of assistants.

◆ Time Management and Organization

You may have the most highly motivated persons working for you, but if they are not organized, work does not get done the way it should be done. As supervisor you are responsible for seeing that the assigned work gets done and that it gets done on time.

Because we cannot manage time, we need to learn to manage ourselves. Everyone has the same number of hours in a day, yet some people accomplish much more than others. The following are some key ideas for getting things done effectively and efficiently: Start each day with a written overview of what needs to be done.

How many patients do you have?

What are their needs?

What assessments, medications, and treatments are needed?

Which patients have appointments? When and where?

Are there physician rounds?

Prioritize your activities.

Do the most important things first.

Identify those activities that *must* be done at a specified time and plan ahead for them.

Identify those things that you must do yourself.

Assign routine activities to your staff.

Plan ahead.

Gather all necessary supplies, but make sure that you leave adequate supplies for the next shift.

Plan your steps.

Concentrate on one thing at a time.

Plan your stops in a logical order.

Write things down.

Carry a notebook or worksheet to note things immediately so that you do not forget.

Identify the departments with which you deal most often, such as the pharmacy and central processing and dispatch department.

List all questions for these departments together so you may settle everything at one time.

Making Assignments

Part of good organization is proper utilization of your nursing assistants. The following are some suggestions:

Make sure that the assigned duties do not exceed the legal limitations or institutional policies.

Consider the strengths and skills of each individual. Match these with the patient's needs.

Provide continuity of care whenever possible.

Consider the physical layout of your unit. Save time by clustering assignments whenever possible.

Do not play favorites. Keep work assignments as fair as possible.

Try various staffing techniques. Use pairs or teams to cover groups of patients.

Problem Employees

Most of the staff whom you supervise will be dependable, conscientious, and hardworking. Unfortunately, it is likely that you may encounter some employees who have serious behavior or attitude problems. Problem employees present risks to patient safety and undermine morale of the more responsible workers. These difficult employees must be handled in a professional manner to avoid untoward legal ramifications. Depending on the nature and severity of the disruption, a situation may require immediate action or may require long-term follow-up. For example, situations related to patient abuse or use of illegal substances are serious and must be addressed immediately, but situations related to punctuality or demeanor are usually less critical and may be handled over a period of time.

Each institution should have due process guidelines that are designed to resolve situations involving problem persons. This process should be explained to employees at all levels at the time of hire so that no questions arise when the process is needed.

Basic rules for dealing with problem individuals include the following:

Stay calm; do not lose your temper or overreact

Take whatever actions are needed to protect patient safety, including removing the disruptive person from patient contact.

Inform the person that the disruptive behavior is not acceptable in the workplace. Criticism, corrections, and reprimands should be given in private. If witnesses are required, other supervisory personnel should be involved, not peers of the problem employee.

Notify the supervising registered nurse of the problem promptly. Facts should be communicated verbally and in writing.

Begin documentation at the first sign of possible problems.

Document the specific facts, not your perceptions. Use accurate descriptions of events and direct quotes from involved parties just as with charting.

◆ Values Clarification Exercises

For each exercise number a sheet of paper from 1 to 10, or use ten slips of paper. Write the first ten thoughts or statements that come to mind. Do not judge the ideas as you write them down. After you have written ten different replies to each exercise, go back and rank them in order going from that which best describes you or is most important (rank this number 1) and continue to that which least describes you or is least important (rank this number 10).

Exercise 1

Who am I?   Importance

1. _____   _____

2. _____   _____

3. _____   _____

4. _____   _____

5. _____   _____

6. _____   _____

7. _____   _____

8. _____   _____

9. _____   _____

10. _____   _____

(Set up is the same for remaining exercises as for Exercise 1.)

Exercise 2   Things I like to do

Exercise 3   People with whom I like to spend time

Exercise 4   Things I like about myself

Exercise 5   Things I would like to improve

Exercise 6   When I am angry I . . .

Exercise 7   When someone is supervising me, I want them to . . .

◆ Listening Skills Quiz

Directions: Read the following questions, and then rate yourself accordingly.

4 points if always
3 points if almost always
2 points if rarely
1 point if never

_____ 1. Do I allow the speaker to finish a complete thought before asking questions or interrupting?

_____ 2. Do I listen between the lines and look for nonverbal cues or hidden meanings?

_____ 3. Do I listen without becoming upset if the speaker's point of view is different from my own?

_____ 4. Do I write down important facts or information so that I do not forget?

_____ 5. If I am interrupted, do I stop and give my total attention to the speaker?

_____ 6. If I have been given complicated directions, do I repeat them to the speaker for verification before ending the conversation?

_____ 7. Do I listen carefully, even if I think the speaker is less intelligent or less experienced than I am?

_____ 8. Do I avoid becoming distracted when someone is speaking to me?

_____ 9. I try to understand and empathize with the speaker.

_____ 10. I ask questions if I am not sure I understand what the speaker says.

Scoring: If you score above 32, you have excellent listening skills. If your score is 27 to 31, you are an above-average listener. If your score is 22 to 26, you need to practice listening skills, and if your score is 21 or less you need to work on your listening skills. Look at the areas marked rarely or never. These are good places to start making changes.

◆ _Study Helps_

1. List two tasks performed by high level managers.
2. What is involved in supervision?
3. Define leadership and supervision.
4. Define a group.
5. List some of your strengths and weaknesses.
6. Describe how the licensed practical nurse can effectively listen to ancillary personnel.
7. List three reasons for using written communication.
8. List four ways you can motivate your staff.
9. List three ways you can more effectively manage time.
10. List three styles of leadership and briefly describe each.

Bibliography

Abruzzese RS: Nursing staff development: strategies for success in the 90s, St Louis, 1991, Mosby.

Cribbin JJ: *Leadership,* New York, 1981, AMACOM Book Division.

Douglass, LM: *The effective nurse: leader and manager,* St Louis, 1992, Mosby.

Ellis JR, Nowlis EA: *Nursing: a human needs approach,* ed 4, Boston, 1989, Houghton-Mifflin.

Haimann T, Hilgert RL: *Supervision: concepts and practices of management,* ed 4, Cincinnati, 1987, South-Western Publishing.

Hill SS, Howlett HA: *Success in practical nursing,* Philadelphia, 1993, WB Saunders.

Holle ML: *Introduction to leadership and management in nursing,* Monterey, Calif, 1987, Jones and Bartlett.

Moloney MM: *Leadership in nursing,* St Louis, 1979, Mosby.

Ring MK, Bond D: *Gerontology and leadership skills for nurses,* 1991, Delmar.

Steele SM, Harmon VM: *Values clarification in nursing,* ed 2, Norwalk, Conn, 1983, Appleton-Century-Crofts.

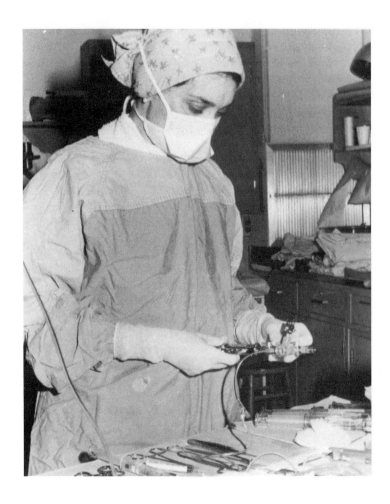

Objectives

At the completion of this chapter the student practical nurse will be able to:

◆ Discuss self-evaluation.

◆ List important benefits when seeking employment.

◆ Develop a personal budget plan.

◆ Discuss ways in which a nurse may continue her education.

◆ Differentiate between BSN, ADN, and diploma nursing programs.

9 Entry into Practice and Continuing Education

In all probability you will seek and accept a position of employment in nursing even before you have received your license to practice. However, doing so is permissible because the state board of nursing allows you to work 30 to 90 days, depending on the individual state, while you are applying for and receiving your licensure.

Your choice of employment should be considered carefully. You should be familiar with the fields open to the licensed practical nurse. You should know yourself. Self-knowledge includes knowing your abilities and skills, likes and dislikes, strengths and weaknesses. You must also consider the personal and professional satisfaction that you hope to gain from this specific type of job.

◆ Self-Evaluation

Self-evaluation means examining one's assets as well as one's defects. Two points that should always be included are self-sufficiency and self-confidence. The rule of success is "have a positive attitude and know yourself."

You cannot function well in every area. Your likes and dislikes influence your performance. Your instructors can assist you greatly in selecting a suitable and enjoyable field in which to work. The instructors, through learning and experience, are in a position to evaluate your capabilities. Through periodic conferences and counseling they aim to help you strengthen your weak areas and develop your strong areas. Listen to suggestions from those who know you and want to help you. Perhaps they can open new horizons that you have never considered. Accept criticism gracefully and profit from it. You do not have to agree with it, but try to be realistic and honest with yourself. A careful study of your personality, your abilities, and your achievements in nursing helps you to decide the area of nursing for which you are best suited. Your aim is to fulfill the needs of others, but in doing so you must fulfill certain needs of your own.

◆ Position Analysis

You will not find a perfect job. Each one has advantages and disadvantages. The selection of a field of nursing is a major decision. Previously, licensed practical nurses

127

had few areas from which to choose; today the fields they may enter are many. Remember that every field does not appeal to everyone. Humans were not created with the same likes and dislikes, the same personalities, or the same beliefs. If interests vary, then the type of work suited to each person also varies.

A quick look at some of the advantages and disadvantages in the major areas available to the practical nurse today may prove beneficial.

Finding a Position

There is a shortage of nursing personnel in some areas. You may discover available positions through word of mouth, hospitals, schools, agencies, or advertisements. Because the qualifications for the job, the benefits, and the possible drawbacks may be easily distorted, never presume. Know the full responsibilities, the philosophy, the salary, and the hours. Ask to see the personnel policies and read them carefully. Arrange for a personal interview before you make any commitments.

Evaluation of Positions

When evaluating positions, you must consider many factors. Some of these factors include salary, hours and days, vacation and sick leave, maternity leave, adoptive leave, child care, leave of absence and holiday time, transportation, reputation of employer, promotional opportunities, laundry and uniforms, meals, in-service education, environmental factors, and insurance benefits. Each of these factors is discussed briefly. Ask yourself questions concerning each of the following considerations.

Salary. Salary is important, but it is not everything. Other factors such as opportunities for advancement, experience, further educational opportunities, and incremental increases in salary after you have proved your worth are also important. Sometimes high salaries are offered because the position requires more responsibility than you as a practical nurse are prepared to assume. High salaries are often used as an enticement to secure nurses for needed positions. Although a good salary is important, equally important is a good benefits package. *Both* factors should be considered when seeking employment.

Hours and days. Are you planning to work full time or part time? What hours are entailed? Must you rotate shifts? How many weekends must you work? How are you compensated for evening or night shifts?

Vacation and sick leave. Two benefits are vacation and sick time. Ask yourself these questions: Is a time for sick leave and vacation provided? If so, how long is it? Is it with or without pay? Does it increase with the length of service? Does the hospital give a discount for room and medications if needed by the employee?

Maternity leave. Does the institution provide time off for the birth of a baby? If so, how long? May the time be extended if the physician orders?

Adoptive leave. Does the institution provide time off for the mother of an adopted child? How long?

Child care. Does the institution provide child care for its employees? If so, what are the hours, the cost, and the ages of children accepted? Are the people employed to care for the children dependable, knowledgeable, and caring? Is the facility near a part of the hospital to which you are applying?

Leave of absence and holiday time. How many holidays are provided each year? Is a leave of absence granted? If so, which conditions are necessary to obtain this leave? Is it with or without pay? What is the employee's status on returning from a leave?

Transportation. How far is the institution from where you live? Do you have a car? If not, is adequate bus service available? Can you really depend on another person for transportation? Will rotation of shifts cause transportation problems? Are parking facilities free, safe, and adequate?

Reputation of employer. Does the employer or institution have a good reputation? Is it known for its high standards? Is it accredited by professional organizations? Is the turnover of nursing personnel high? If so, investigate this turnover thoroughly.

Promotional opportunities. Are periodic raises given? Are they automatic, or do they depend on a personal evaluation of your performance? What is the top salary that is available to a licensed practical nurse? What length of time is normally required to obtain it? To what position can a practical nurse be promoted?

Laundry and uniforms. Must you supply or launder your own uniforms, or does the institution provide this service? Which types of uniforms are allowed? Which uniform regulations exist for the employee?

Meals. Do the employees receive free meals while on duty? If not, do they receive a discount? Are coffee breaks provided? If so, how many are there and for what length of time? Does the institution have a cafeteria or suitable place in which to eat?

In-service education. Is the institution education-oriented? Is there an orientation program? Is there a program for in-service education? Which areas are covered by the program? How often are these programs given?

Tuition reimbursement. Does the institution offer tuition reimbursement to employees desiring to continue their education outside the hospital? Must the courses be job-related? Is this benefit available on employment or after a time of employment? How much of the tuition cost is reimbursed to the employee? If this education is in a college, how many credit hours may the employee take in one semester? Must the employee achieve a certain grade to be reimbursed? How long may the employee take to achieve her educational goal?

Environmental factors. Is the institution neat, clean, cheerful, and progressive? Is it equipped with the up-to-date machinery needed to render quality nursing care to the patient? What is the morale of the employees?

Insurance benefits. Does the institution make provisions for group or individual plans? Which types of insurance plans does it offer—life, liability, salary continuance, medical, and dental plans? What is the coverage of these insurance plans? Does the employer carry compensation insurance for accidents or sickness of the employee?

If the institution does not provide liability insurance, the practical nurse should think in terms of securing it to cover claims and costs of legal counsel that may arise from negligence or damage or both occurring while giving care. With liability insurance you are covered even if the claim is false, groundless, or fraudulent. The premiums are deductible from your federal income tax. Group premium rates are available through most state licensed practical nurse associations. The constantly increasing number of lawsuits involving alleged malpractice now makes liability insurance a necessity.

Credit union. Does the institution have a credit union? Is the employee able to make a deposit in a credit union account through a payroll deduction? How much interest is paid to the investor? How much interest is charged by the credit union for a personal loan?

Pension plan. Who is eligible? Does the employer pay the premium, or is a portion deducted from the employee's paycheck? What percentage of base pay does the employee receive on retirement? Is there a compulsory retirement age?

◇   ◇   ◇

After you have thoroughly evaluated these factors, you must decide whether the position is suitable for you personally and economically.

◆ Applying for a Position

After you have carefully considered the position you want and its various aspects, you must apply for the position. This is done by written application or by personal interview. If you are applying by written application, keep the essentials of good letter writing in mind. Use white paper. Never use colored or lined paper. Either type your letter or write it in ink. Use the proper salutation. Avoid using the phrase "to whom it may concern." Use proper English, spell correctly, and use correct punctuation. Provide margins on your letter. Do not enclose photographs, diplomas, or references unless specified. When you wish to use a person's name as a reference, ask the person for permission to use his name. Be sure to thank him for the reference. A sample letter is shown on p.131.

The following points should be included in your letter:
1. State the purpose of the letter and the position for which you are applying.
2. Give the source of information concerning the job. This may be through advertisement, a previous employer, or a recommendation from someone.
3. Give your qualifications and past experiences. They help the employer judge whether you have the proper preparation for the job.
4. You may request an application blank or an appointment for an interview.
5. Express your appreciation for the employer's consideration.
6. Sign your full name and give your address and phone number.

◆ **Sample Letter of Application**

400 E. 35th St.
Chicago, IL 60612

February 20,
1993

Ms. Margaret Ames
Director of Nurses
St. Simeon Health Center
Centreville, IL 60654

Dear Ms. Ames:

A previous employer has told me of your need for a licensed practical nurse to work the evening shift on weekends.

I would appreciate your considering me for this position. I am a graduate of the Boone County Practical Nursing Program in Clinton, Iowa. For the past 10 years I have worked as a licensed practical nurse on a medical unit. I have functioned as a team leader, a medicine nurse, and, on occasion, a charge nurse.

May I have an appointment to speak with you at your earliest convenience? You may write to me at the above address or call me at (312) 459-8280 after 6 P.M.

Sincerely,

Dorothy White, LPN

Application Form

Most employers request that you complete an application form before you are interviewed. These forms may vary with the institution, but all forms essentially contain the following:

Your name (include your maiden name if married)
Address
Telephone number
Social Security number
License number
Education
Previous places of employment, their addresses, and the length of time employed in each place
Reference names and addresses
Job for which you are applying

An application form aids the employer in eliminating the applicants who do not possess the desired qualifications for the position and provides the employer with necessary information. It becomes an important part of the employer's file if the applicant is hired, or it may be kept on file for future openings requiring these qualifications.

Interview

Always make an appointment in advance for an interview. This may be done by letter or by phone. This shows consideration for the employer, and it also assures you of a specific time and date.

The purpose of the interview is twofold. It provides the employer with the opportunity to determine whether you qualify for the position, and it gives you the opportunity to evaluate the job in terms of your needs and expectations. Therefore the interviewer and you have two objectives in mind: giving and receiving information. Each is evaluating the other.

Be sure to be on time, preferably a few minutes early. Try to be composed and relaxed. Make sure that you are properly groomed and dressed. Know the name of the person who is to interview you. Never chew gum! Do not smoke unless invited to do so. Remain standing until you are told to be seated. Remain poised and alert. Listen carefully and answer as simply and honestly as possible. Neither exaggerate nor underestimate your abilities. When asked about your previous experiences, state them in a matter-of-fact manner.

Before you accept the position, be sure that it is the position you are seeking and desire. Know the salary, the personnel policies, and the duties and responsibilities that will be expected of you. If several people are applying for the same position, ask the interviewer when he plans to make a decision. If you do not believe that the position is suited to you, then express these feelings to the interviewer. Thank him for his time and interest and leave.

◆ Retaining Your Position

To retain your position you must accept its imposed responsibilities. This includes reporting on and off duty, notifying the proper person if you are ill, and giving your employer sufficient time to secure a replacement. You should understand your duties and show interest in their performance. Be willing to give the best of your abilities and show your worth to others. Above all, try to find happiness and success in your job. All jobs have good and bad points, but usually the good points outweigh the bad. Do not change jobs too frequently. Recommendations are better the longer you retain a certain position. Never walk away from your duties or responsibilities. Remember that in return for your services, the employer has contracted to pay you a definite salary with certain fringe benefits. He has a right to demand a good day's work in return for a just salary. If you take a strong character and a good personality to a new position, you will advance personally and professionally. Joy in what you are doing, together with sufficient preparation and knowledge, helps you to give quality nursing care to the patient and to be a pleasant coworker to members of the team.

Advancement

Advancement may result from additional preparation or additional experience. It may be made by learning the position more thoroughly and by assuming new and greater responsibilities. Advancements, together with the difficulties and obstacles that they bring, stimulate interest and enthusiasm. They are usually based on a person's qualifications, behavior, performance, and preparation.

Resignation

If you decide to resign your position in a certain institution, think the matter over carefully. After you have reached your decision, give at least a 2-week notice, depending on personnel policies of the institution. Never walk off duty without previous notice. In rare circumstances the notice may be shortened or omitted with legitimate reasons. A sample letter of resignation is shown below. Some institutions have resignation forms to be filled in by the employee. These forms include the date of termination, reasons for leaving, and evaluation of employment. Make arrangements for your final paycheck. Take the resignation form or letter to your employer in person if possible. Leave the institution in good standing; keep any feelings of resentment to yourself. Remember that future recommendations depend on your manner and procedure of resignation.

Dismissal

Reasons for dismissal may be dishonesty, insubordination, unlawful or wrong actions, or failure to observe rules and regulations. In these instances you may be dis-

---

◆ Sample Letter of Resignation

March 12, 1993

Mr. Jerome Bigh
Director of Nurses
Faith Hospital
4950 Towne Rd.
St. Louis, MO 65482

Dear Mr. Bigh:

I am resigning my position as charge nurse on the third floor medical unit. My husband and I are moving to Florida to be nearer to our aging parents.

I am giving the required 2-week notice. My last day of work will be March 26, 1993.

I have enjoyed my work here for the past 6 years. I am grateful to you for your kindness, assistance, and encouragement.

Sincerely,

Jane Braun, LPN

charged without notice and may forfeit any benefits such as holidays, sick leave, or vacation time. You will be paid in full for the days worked. In most cases of dismissal a 2-week notice is given. If you believe that the dismissal is unfair, you have the right to appeal to the director of personnel. The director has the duty to hear and review your case and make the final decision. If dismissal occurs during the probationary period or from a temporary position, you are not entitled to any benefits. Dismissal policies may vary in different types of institutions.

Failure

Why do some people fail in their positions? Sometimes failure may be attributed to character limitations. These limitations may include poor interpersonal relationships, lack of cooperation, insincerity, and jealousy. Other causes of failure may be lack of knowledge regarding the position, inability to deal with patients and coworkers, or failure to demonstrate one's abilities. Every employee has basic needs that must be fulfilled. Recognition and acceptance are important needs that must be met. If they are not met, job dissatisfaction and insecurity may result.

The position you choose must meet your needs, and you must meet the needs of the job. If the position you choose fails to bring you satisfaction, you will be unhappy and your behavior and patient care will soon reflect this. If you are unprepared for the position you choose, you will soon experience frustration and will be overwhelmed by the expectations of your employer. What can you do? There are two alternatives: change positions or do something to correct the problem. If you feel the job does not meet your needs and you can do nothing to effect a change, resignation is your alternative. If you feel educationally unprepared, consider continuing your education. A wise person never stops learning, and learning may be attained in many ways: learning on the job, in-service programs in the hospital, attending conventions and workshops, reading professional journals, watching educational television programs, or taking regular or extension courses in a graduate school, college, or junior college. The most important factor is your willingness to change and to learn. Regardless of the educational programs made available to you, they are of little or no value unless you want to learn.

◆ Budget

Your economic status determines the way you live. Therefore the wise spending of money necessitates a budget.

Suggested Budget Plan

A budget or spending plan is a tool. It helps you manage money wisely and attain your financial goals. A budget helps you eliminate inefficient spending and gives you more for your money. To be workable, your budget must be tailored for you. It should be adapted to your needs and income. Preparing a budget for yourself takes planning, and following a budget requires determination.

The types of forms and systems for handling money are many, but the principle is still the same. You must list your definite obligations and in this way discover how much money you must put aside to meet these outlays. From this you can estimate how much money you have to spend and how much you can save.

◆ **Sample Budget**

FEBRUARY

Your Net Monthly Income: $2200.00	Budget amount	Actual amount
Necessary fixed-expense items		
Rent payment	500	500
Auto payment	200	200
School loan	50	50
Other loan	25	25
Health insurance	65	65
Auto insurance	75	75
Church contribution	100	100
	1015	1015
Necessary variable-expense items		
Utility{md}electric	65	50
Utility{md}water	20	25
Utility{md}gas	35	35
Telephone bill	40	35
Auto gas	30	70
Food{md}groceries	200	225
Child care	50	85
	440	525
Optional fixed-expense items		
Cable television	25	25
Life insurance	50	50
Disability insurance	25	25
Savings	200	200
	300	300
Optional variable-expense items		
Food{md}dining out	50	65
Clothing	60	75
Entertainment	50	60
Cash	40	50
	200	250
TOTALS	1955	2090

Miscellaneous (difference between monthly total amount earned and total monthly amount spent)

	245	110

In its simplest form a money management plan consists of four sets of figures. It makes little difference with which set you begin. For convenience the sets are assigned a certain order and labeled Steps 1, 2, 3, and 4. The plan shown in the box on p. 135 is based on a monthly system.

Your Income

Write down how much money you expect to receive for 1 month. Be certain to include all types of income. When listing wages and salaries, write down what you actually receive, or your net income. Do not include withholding taxes and other deductions. This does not mean, however, that it is safe for you to ignore payroll deductions when you establish your program. If a deduction is for hospitalization or group life insurance, it is payment toward your protection. If it is for purchasing a savings bond or pension, it is payment toward your savings. Some payroll deductions are set by law. Others may be increased or decreased as your situation changes.

Step 1: necessary fixed expense items. Write down all the fixed obligations you have to meet during a 1-month period. Examples of these are rent or mortgage payments, installment payments, life insurance, church contributions, and taxes over and above your payroll taxes. Do not write down expenses you cannot estimate closely; include only fixed obligations or expenses you can estimate closely. Total these items. Each month you must have this amount in the bank or a special fund; when one of your fixed items comes due, pay it from this fund. Once the system is well under way, if your original estimates were correct, there will always be sufficient funds to meet your obligations.

Step 2: necessary variable-expense items. From your monthly income subtract your fixed expenses and determine your day to day expenses. These are food, utilities, transportation, car maintenance, child care, and other such items. To know if your plan will work, you must estimate these items as closely as possible and then check the total with the balance of your monthly income. If the balance is insufficient to cover variable-expense items, you must refigure the provision you made for other items.

Step 3: optional fixed-expense items. These generally cost the same each month. Your savings is included in this step and should be 10% of your monthly income. Consistently setting this amount aside each month gives you security and the ability to achieve a future goal (for example, a new car, home, or vacation).

Step 4: optional variable-expense items. These are items difficult to estimate. They are items purchased or money spent after all fixed expenses are met (for example, dining out and clothing purchases).

Miscellaneous. Do not consider this as savings. It is an emergency fund to be used for expenses not previously estimated (for example, new tires for your car or motor repairs on your car). This is a sum of money to tide you over bad weeks or months.

◆ Continuing Education

In-Service Education

Many hospitals, as well as other places of employment, have in-service education programs. When you secure a new position, the first in-service education that you receive is a program of orientation. If specific procedures must be performed, a series of concentrated classes may follow. An example of an institution using orientation in-service education is a rehabilitation hospital. Although the licensed practical nurse may already be familiar with range of motion exercises, these and other pertinent procedures are reviewed with new personnel.

Each hospital has its own definite nursing care procedures, and personnel are required to follow these techniques rather than those previously learned. This uniformity helps assure safety to patients and personnel. Some institutions provide follow-up classes to keep their employees abreast of current trends in patient care. Other in-service educational programs include special classes in the administration of medicines, operating room techniques, labor and delivery care, and cardiopulmonary resuscitation.

These classes are given on duty time. Since they are offered for the advancement of the employee, you should take advantage of them. You should never need to be forced to attend these classes. Financially it is costly to the institution to offer such programs, but the advances made in nursing care as a result compensate for this cost. If you fail to attend these programs, it is a loss to you, your patients, and the institution where you are employed.

Conventions and Workshops

Conventions and workshops are held locally, statewide, regionally, and nationally in a variety of forms. They may be offered or sponsored by alumni organizations; state organizations; the National Association for Practical Nurse Education and Service, Inc.; or the National Federation of Licensed Practical Nurses. In addition, 1- to 3-day workshops are offered by the American Heart Association and the National Cancer Society. You cannot expect to attend every convention offered. However, if the hospital does not make provision for its employees to attend these conventions or workshops, you may attend them on your day off or request days of your vacation time for this purpose. Programs offered on a local level are usually of shorter duration, and attendance presents fewer problems. You have heard many times that "nothing stands still." Either a person progresses or regresses. The same is true in the nursing profession. Every day new advances, techniques, and methods of nursing care are being developed. Unless you become familiar with these developments and adopt them according to the policies of your hospital or institution, you gradually become less efficient, and your activities are limited.

Professional Journals and Publications

Reading articles from professional journals is valuable. Some journals are published especially for the licensed practical nurse, including the *Journal of Practical Nursing, Journal of Nursing Care,* and state and local publications.

The *Journal of Practical Nursing* is published by the National Association for Practical Nurse Education and Service, Inc., 254 West 31st Street, New York, NY 10001. It is a monthly publication that keeps you informed about national activities in your practical nursing group. It contains articles on nursing topics, coming events, available positions, new books and pamphlets, and activities occurring in the various states.

The *Journal of Nursing Care* is published by Health Science Division, Technomic Publishing Co., Inc., 265 Post Road West, Westport, CT 06880. It is a monthly publication that contains information about and activities of the National Federation of Licensed Practical Nurses. It includes reports from committees representing practical nursing, progress of practical nursing education programs, and any announcements the national headquarters desires to convey to its state or local members.

You should become familiar with your state and local nursing publications. They are usually in the form of bulletins, journals, or magazines. They contain valuable information concerning the officers of your state and local divisions of your organization, plus events, programs, achievements, and happenings in your immediate vicinity.

Because procedures and techniques may change with new developments in medicine, you should maintain proficiency by periodically reading new texts and references by leading publishers in nursing. New publications are advertised in most professional journals.

Post-licensure Programs

Post-licensure programs may be very beneficial to a licensed practical nurse who does not feel adequately prepared to assume responsibilities in a particular field. Some instructors and administrative personnel believe that it is wise for a new nurse to work for 6 months to 1 year in a general hospital to gain necessary experience. During student days some practical experience is acquired, but theory is emphasized. After graduation limited theoretical knowledge is gained, and emphasis is placed on practical experience. After a year spent in a general hospital, the licensed practical nurse has sufficient background to specialize in one particular area and is equipped with a varied background sufficient for functioning smoothly and efficiently.

Before enrolling in a post-licensure program, investigate to see if it is an accredited program. You must consider all factors involved. Some of these include length of time, cost, and living expenses needed. Some programs may mean living away from home or even in another state.

The post-licensure programs available may be found in monthly publications from your local, state, or national organizations. They list the courses offered, the dates, and the locations where they are offered.

Refresher Courses

Nursing organizations. Refresher courses are offered by the home nursing school, local organizations, or state and national nursing organizations. They are offered to those wishing to bring themselves up to date with current trends in nursing care. The length of the course may vary with individual groups, material being taught, and different instructors. Many schools of practical nursing are now offering courses to their alumni and other interested licensed practical nurses. The most commonly offered course is administration of medicines.

Local branches of the American National Red Cross offer courses such as first aid, cardiopulmonary resuscitation, swimming, and water safety. The procedures taught in these courses are current and serve as valuable aids to nursing and nonnursing persons.

Television. Television is being used to give extension courses in useful subjects for continuing education. Many of these programs award certificates on the completion of the course. Notices of these programs may be found in the daily newspaper and television guides and through your employing hospital or agency. These notices are often posted on the bulletin board or announced at various meetings.

Registered Nursing Programs

Bachelor of science degree in nursing (BSN) program. The BSN program is one that consists of approximately 4 years of university or college training. At the completion of the program the graduate qualifies to take a licensing examination to become a registered nurse and also receives a bachelor of science degree in nursing from the university or college.

In this program, nursing theory and skills are incorporated with managerial theory and skills. Stress is placed on understanding the entire patient in depth. This understanding includes physical, social, psychological, religious, and economic aspects. The program delves deeply into human behavior and methods of effectively coping with problem situations.

The student learns the theory and skills of nursing and is given opportunities to function in all capacities of a registered nurse under proper supervision.

This program tends to mature the student in all aspects. The nurse develops socially, physically, and psychologically. This educational program provides the individual with the poise and competency required of a registered nurse.

Associate degree nursing (ADN) program. The ADN program is offered by community colleges, colleges, and universities. It is designed to prepare the student to assume the responsibilities related to direct patient care as a member of the health team in hospitals and in community health agencies.

In some areas the curriculum has been revised to incorporate the career ladder concept. The first-year curriculum includes the minimum requirements necessary for the student to become eligible for licensure as a licensed practical nurse. On the successful completion of the entire curriculum, the student is eligible to take the state board of nursing examination for licensure as a registered nurse.

The clinical experience is limited in this program. Emphasis is placed on educational background. Clinical experience is given in several hospitals.

After this 2-year program an internship program may prove valuable to the new graduate. This program may rotate the new graduate through areas of a general hospital, providing her with ample opportunities to integrate theory with clinical experience.

Diploma program in nursing. The diploma program is offered by a private institution or organization. It combines nursing theory and skills. The curriculum is planned over a specific period to give the student sufficient time in all major areas of nursing. This amount of time enables the student to learn procedures and disease conditions thoroughly in each area. It rotates the student through every job performed by the registered nurse. Emphasis is placed equally on theory and clinical experience. It prepares a bedside nurse, team leader, treatment nurse, or medication nurse. At the completion of the course the graduate is qualified to take the licensure examination to become a registered nurse and is awarded a diploma from the nursing school.

◇   ◇   ◇

Regardless of the type of nursing program you choose, the fundamental objective of each is quality nursing care. Each deals with patients, their families, and other members of the health team. As a nurse you must develop all your potentials. This means that you meet not only your own needs but also those of the patient. As a licensed practical nurse you have responsibilities to yourself, your patients, your nursing organization, and your community. Nursing is a vocation of service. Your uniform is the badge showing the vocation you have chosen; wear it proudly as you serve others.

◆ *Study Helps*

1. What factors should be considered when applying for employment?
2. In which way does a budget help you to remain financially stable?
3. Describe the demeanor of an individual applying for a position.
4. What opportunities are available for continuing your education after licensure?
5. Which types of in-service programs do most institutions offer?
6. Of what importance are conventions and workshops?
7. Differentiate among the following: BSN programs, ADN programs, and diploma programs.
8. What type of vocation is nursing?

Bibliography

Berhard LA, Walsh M: *Leadership: the key to the professionalization of nursing,* ed 2, St Louis, 1990, Mosby.
Kurzen CR: *Contemporary practical/vocational nursing,* Philadelphia, 1989, JB Lippincott.
McCloskey JC, Grace HK: *Current issues in nursing,* ed 3, St Louis, 1990, Mosby.

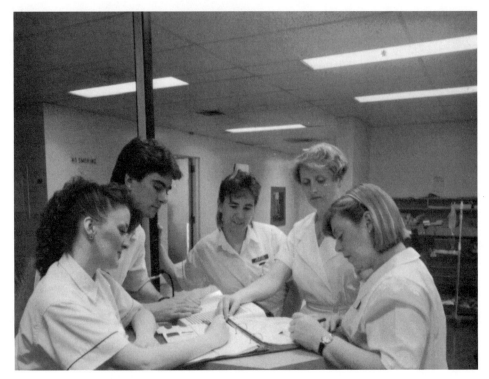

Courtesy Prime Communications Consultants, St John's Lane Photographics Ltd, St John's and the Association of Registered Nurses of Newfoundland

Objectives

At the completion of this chapter the student practical nurse will be able to:

◆ Discuss the purposes of three types of health clinics.

◆ List at least five areas in which the licensed practical nurse may find employment.

◆ Discuss the advantages and disadvantages of working in five different areas of employment.

◆ Discuss the licensed practical nurse's role in public relations.

$\diamondsuit$ 10 Practicing the Vocation

Because of the ever-changing supply and demand for nurses, today's licensed practical nurse has options that were not available to nurses who completed programs 10 or more years ago. Licensed practical nurses earn good salaries, have insurance and sick benefits, earn vacation time, receive tuition assistance, have flexible work schedules, and find employment in a variety of health care settings.

A clear understanding of each setting may help you in making your future choice in the specific area that is of interest to you.

◆ Licensed Practical Nurse in the General Hospital

Many opportunities are available in the hospital to use your abilities as a licensed practical nurse to the fullest extent. If giving direct care to the patient is your greatest interest, then working as a bedside nurse may meet your needs. Often by working directly with the patient, you become the most important person in the hospital to him. You spend longer periods of time with him than any of the other personnel. You can help meet the patient's needs by accurately reporting them to the team leader or head nurse, who in turn reports them to the physician. Your duties depend on hospital policies and your training and work record. You should be familiar with the hospital's job description for the position for which you have been employed. A careful study of this job description shows your clearly defined role in the health team.

The 8-hour tour of duty that you follow is usually 7 AM to 3:30 PM, 3 PM to 11:30 PM, or 11 PM to 7:30 AM. It may be any one of these, or it may be a combination of all of these. Usually your days off are rotated so that everyone has equal opportunity for holidays and weekends. Before accepting a position, you should check and know the hospital's policies concerning tours of duty. This helps you make previous arrangements so that you can follow duty schedules.

There are many advantages to working in a hospital. Employment is steady, and most hospitals have good personnel policies. Ordinarily you may choose any one of the specific areas in the hospital that are available. These areas include obstetrics, pediatrics, general medicine, surgery, and psychiatry. They may also include one of the specialties such as the operating room.

The nurse chooses to work in the clinical area that best fits her personality, skills, and needs. For instance, did you ever notice the typical nurse in a surgical area? Usually the operating room nurse is quick-moving, energetic, and adept with machines and procedures. The surgical area always has the high dramatic element: the psychological preparation before surgery and the first critical postoperative hours with much pain and possible complications are usually followed by dramatic daily improvement. Nausea, distention, and inability to void are common postoperative problems. Various drainage tubes, chest tube bottles, tracheostomy care, and dressing changes create a challenging environment and warrant an observing practitioner skilled at working in such a situation. The surgical nurse may communicate more with actions than words.

Contrast the surgery patient to the patient in a coronary care unit whose wound is not visible although he is possibly in more imminent danger of death. A coronary patient requires a nurse with a particular emotional makeup, depth of knowledge, and the ability to recognize subtle signs of changing condition. This nurse must be able to recognize a multitude of monitor patterns and be able to act quickly and expertly without alarming the patient. It is a demanding role that requires a certain balance and type of personality.

Medical nursing is challenging because of the subtlety of signs, changing conditions, and the necessity of sustaining the spirit of the patient who has long, often chronic, recurring exacerbations of his illness. It requires a nurse who has great empathy and endurance.

A good psychiatric nurse must have a stable emotional makeup. Because so much of psychiatric nursing involves active therapy for the depressed and apathetic patient, this is not an area for the overly empathetic and emotional nurse. Although physical expenditure is small in psychiatric nursing, mental strain and tension are great.

Some nurses like to function in extremely active areas with little time for rest and relaxation, such as in the emergency room, delivery room, or treatment room. The night shift in the emergency room may deal with two minor conditions one night and perhaps twenty critical conditions the next night, including a cardiac arrest and five admissions. In all these areas, experiences are varied and offer many opportunities for learning.

While working in a general hospital, you find opportunities to advance your knowledge and your skills. The duties you may perform as a licensed practical nurse are regulated by the state board of nursing as well as by the individual hospital. Regardless of your preparation and experience, you may perform only those procedures and functions legislated for the licensed practical nurse.

All practical nurses working in specialized areas need postlicensure training to better qualify them for the role they are expected to fulfill. In a hospital, this may include a basic dysrhythmia course or an intravenous therapy course; in a nursing home, courses in management and leadership; and in home health care, courses that help the nurse better develop assessment skills and interpersonal relationships.

The community, the hospital, your professional organizations, and your patients depend on you to continue your education through in-service programs, courses, or readings. Only by keeping abreast of nursing and its newest procedures and theories are you able to function adequately.

◆ Licensed Practical Nurse in Occupational Health

Most industrial plants are required to have health programs for their employees. These programs are under the supervision of a physician and registered nurse, often with a licensed practical nurse working as an assistant. If you choose to work in industry, you must know the duties performed by each level of employee, ranging from the unskilled laborer to top administrator. This information is needed to help plan and carry out necessary accident prevention programs. Because you work closely with employer and employee, you must understand the overall industry and its functions to meet their personal and health needs.

Many industries require preemployment physicals, as well as yearly physicals. For particular reasons some industries may require these physicals more often. Most industries that provide health programs and employ nurses to staff these programs also have an emergency program. You may administer first aid as indicated. You may be required to test vision and hearing. You may be expected to keep health records current on all employees. Your job responsibilities may vary greatly, depending on the industry and its specific type of work.

The hours are usually desirable. In some places you may be asked to rotate shifts. Salaries are higher than those paid in institutional nursing.

In this field of nursing you must have patience, understanding, observational skills, and current first-aid techniques and principles. You must possess organizational skills and neatness in keeping records. You must be able to adjust to all types of situations and people.

◆ Licensed Practical Nurse in Public Health

Today public health nursing accepts the licensed practical nurse. In this area you may be active in either local or state programs. As a visiting nurse you represent a voluntary community agency. As a public health nurse you represent an official health agency.

Most agencies provide means of transportation, which may be in the form of a car, bus fare, or reimbursement for gasoline and depreciation of your own car. The areas are mapped in such a way that you do not usually have to travel too extensively. This means that you can provide care to more patients in less time. Your work, however, is not limited to rendering care to patients in their homes. It also includes work in school health activities and various types of clinics.

Some of the school health services that are rendered are as follows:
1. Appraising health of faculty and students through
   a. Physical examinations
   b. Dental examinations
   c. Psychological examinations
2. Counseling students, parents, and faculty with regard to health problems
3. Follow-up services in securing correction of remedial defects

4. Assistance in discovery and education of handicapped children
5. Prevention and control of communicable diseases, including immunizations
6. Provision of emergency service in case of injury or sudden illness

Following are some types of clinics:

1. *Maternal and child health clinics* attempt to improve the hygienic conditions of maternity, infancy, and childhood and offer prenatal and infant care, including health education.
2. *Crippled children clinics* investigate the prevalence of crippling conditions and provide supplementary aid in rehabilitation of the children affected.
3. *Mental health clinics* help assess the extent of mental hygiene services needed in a community, carry on educational programs in this area, and offer assistance to affected persons.

Other services rendered to the public include prevention, detection, and treatment of communicable and social diseases.

If you are interested in working in the field of public health, the first and most basic qualification that you must possess is the ability to accept and work easily with all types of people. This does not mean doing everything for them but rather teaching them to help themselves.

As a licensed practical nurse you are supervised by a registered nurse. Your assignment is made according to your nursing abilities and your personality. You must know or learn the area to which you are assigned. You must be alert and observant. You must be capable of making accurate decisions in accordance with your position in nursing. The workweek usually consists of an 8-hour day, 5 days a week, with holidays and weekends free. Salaries are comparable to those paid in institutions.

The challenges, variety of people and situations, and ideal working hours entice many licensed practical nurses to enter this field of nursing.

◆ Licensed Practical Nurse in Private Duty Nursing

As a private duty nurse you may care for your patient wherever the patient desires. This may be in the home, the hospital, or while traveling abroad or in the United States. In this field you are given the opportunity to know your patient and his family better. You are expected to meet the total needs of the patient. This includes rendering bedside care if needed, showering him with attention, and catering to his every whim and fancy unless contraindicated. You accept not only the patient when doing private duty nursing but also his family. Many times the patient's problems become your problems. Teaching the patient and his family may be one of your chief functions.

When doing private duty nursing, you are legally responsible for your own actions. If you should experience any doubt about an order or procedure, obtain clarification from the physician before carrying out the order or procedure. Charts must be kept carefully. In a hospital setting use the procedure of the hospital. In the home set up a type of record in which you can list necessary items, such as medications given, vital signs, and the condition of the patient. This home record may be requested by the patient's physician and may be released by you to him. Remember that any narcotics not used must be returned to the physician before you leave the case.

The salary scale set by the licensed practical nurse associations and by the American Nurses' Association is approximately three fourths of the salary of the registered nurse for 8 hours of duty.

The chief problems of a private duty nurse are the irregular assignments and the economic aspects. In private duty nursing there is no certainty of an available case or of payment. However, because today so many demands for private duty nurses are unfilled, the availability of cases presents few problems for the licensed practical nurse. The greater problem centers around payment. The patient is responsible for the payment of the fee even if a member of the family hires the nurse. The family is not legally responsible for the payment of the fee. Therefore fees are occasionally difficult to collect.

If you should choose this field of nursing, it is advisable to remember that you are responsible for the payment of your social security, as well as your federal, state, and city taxes. This means that you must keep continuous, accurate records of your days worked and payments received.

An advantage of private duty nursing is that you may work as many days as you like, or you may not accept a case for as long a period of time as you desire. You are given more freedom and less rigid rules to follow in your workday.

◆ Licensed Practical Nurse in the Nursing Home

The Omnibus Budget Reconciliation Act passed in 1987 mandated that all skilled and intermediate nursing care facilities in rural and urban areas provide 24 hours of nursing care by licensed practical nurses 7 days a week. One registered nurse must also be employed 7 days a week for 8 hours a day. This act, plus Medicare and Medicaid regulations, has increased the demand for practical nurses in nursing homes and will continue to increase the demand.

Caring for the elderly patient in a nursing home is hard work. It may involve overcoming the behavioral and attitudinal barriers of the nurse. Health care workers in a nursing home must reconcile their own conflicts regarding aging, dependency, and death. If the nurse is unable to do this, she cannot assist the older person to maintain a life with dignity and comfort.

The practical nurse employed in a nursing home generally works in a less formal environment, enjoys more stable duty hours, and has a greater opportunity for advancement.

Caring for the older person is different than caring for patients in other age-groups. The elderly face losses related to economic, social, psychological, and biological factors. Disease entities and the elderly person's response to these entities are often atypical. Society, through the media in particular, often negates the cultural values associated with aging.

All these factors make the provision of high quality care to the institutionalized geriatric patient a challenging goal. However, the attainment of this goal provides great professional and personal satisfaction.

◆ Licensed Practical Nurse in Home Health Nursing

The changing demands of the 1990s for cost containment, the economy, an aging population, and technological advances in home care have made it necessary to care for the acutely ill person at home. Home health care may be offered by hospitals, government agencies, or private agencies.

Employment in home health nursing requires a nurse who assumes responsibility for assisting patients to recover from acute illness, provides care for chronic illnesses, maintains the patient who needs ongoing care, and assists the family in the care of a terminally ill patient.

With the Medicare prospective payment for cost containment in the institutional setting, patients are discharged after the allotted payment for the particular illness runs out rather than after a recuperative period. Some patients may come home directly from the intensive care unit.

You are required to work with a wide range of home health care providers. These may include registered nurses, physicians, physical therapists, social workers, home health aides, nutritionists, and speech pathologists.

◆ Licensed Practical Nurse in Other Areas

The licensed practical nurse is employed in fields of nursing other than the areas already mentioned. However, the number of licensed practical nurses in these areas varies. Following are some other fields.

Office Nursing

> *Advantages*
> Covered by Social Security
> Usually have Sundays and most evenings free
> Holidays, vacations, duties, and salaries are determined by the physician
> *Disadvantages*
> Work includes secretarial knowledge and skills

Rehabilitation Nursing

Employment in rehabilitation requires a nurse who assumes responsibility for guiding the patient toward health and independence.

> *Advantages*
> Steady employment
> Less formal environment
> An opportunity to provide good bedside care
> *Disadvantages*
> Frequently faced with greater responsibility than generally, educationally, and technically prepared to assume

Extended Care Facilities

Nursing care of the patient during the intermediate period when he no longer requires hospital care but is not well enough to go home is offered in extended care facilities (ECF).

> *Advantages*
> Steady employment

Holidays, vacations, duties, and salaries are determined by the institution

Greater opportunity for advancement

Disadvantages

Poorer salaries and benefits

Frequently faced with greater responsibility than generally, educationally, and technically prepared to assume

Psychiatric Nursing

Psychiatric nursing requires a mature person (not in years) to handle the responsibilities of the job. This type of nursing may be done in an open ward in a general hospital, outpatient clinic, mental health agency, psychiatric hospital, or institution.

Advantages

Good salary

Advancement in leadership areas

Disadvantages

If federally financed, often poorer standard of patient care and working conditions

Insufficient professional guidance from nursing staff and physician

Hospice Care

Employment in hospice nursing requires a mature person (not necessarily in years) to meet the spiritual, physical, emotional, and social needs of the dying person and his family. This type of nursing may be done in a hospital, another facility, or the patient's home.

Advantages

Steady employment

Less formal environment

Opportunities to provide good bedside care that is concerned with pain relief and comfort measures

Disadvantages

Always caring for dying patients

May travel to more than one home each shift

Government

Civil Service. The licensed practical nurse may work in a Veterans Administration hospital or other government hospital.

Advantages

Good salary

Fringe benefits

Good insurance and retirement plans

Disadvantages

The ratio of nursing personnel to patients is sometimes low

Agency. Agency nurses must be flexible and willing to follow the policies and procedures of many institutions.

Advantages
    May choose days and shifts you want to work
    Good salary
Disadvantages
    Must work in many different institutions
    May not have benefits such as sick leave and insurance included

Armed Services (Army). The army requires the licensed practical nurse to be between 17 and 34 years of age and a United States citizen of high moral and personal qualifications. The nurse must be a graduate of a 1-year practical nursing program and must be currently licensed.
    Advantages
        Patriotic service to country
        Travel
        Varied experiences are usually encountered
        Special rank and pay
        Allowance given for clothing and quarters
        Benefits of education, training, medical and dental care, and survivors' insurance
    Disadvantages
        Varied shifts and often rotating divisions
        Regimented type of life

◆ Licensed Practical Nurse and Public Relations

In your daily work in the nursing field you come into close contact with many classifications of workers. All these workers contribute to the patient's welfare either directly or indirectly. They include the physician, registered nurse, student nurse, and ancillary personnel such as nursing assistant and the other members of the health care team in the hospital. Cooperation, kindness, and friendliness must exist among all workers to create a successful healing environment for the patient.

You also are an important representative of the hospital to your patients and their families.

Physician

The physician is the direct link between the patient and the members of the health care team. His orders should be carried out as written; if you have any doubt concerning their interpretation or accuracy, you should ask the physician in a diplomatic way how the order should be executed, because you are legally liable for your actions. Always be courteous and cooperative. While on duty do not become overly familiar with the physician. Do not ask for free medical service or discuss personal problems with him during working hours. Use the physician's last name when speaking to him.

Inspire the patient by showing confidence in his physician. The patient chose his own physician; therefore this choice should be respected. Never suggest to the patient that he can change physicians or ask for consultation from another physician. If you believe that something should be done about the patient's physician, discuss the matter with your head nurse, who is responsible for the patient's welfare and has had experience in handling this type of situation.

Registered Nurse

In a hospital you will be working under the supervision of a registered nurse, who retains authority because of advanced training and education. The registered nurse and practical nurse, together with other ancillary personnel, work as a team providing optimum patient care. Much can be accomplished on a busy nursing unit and in a lesser amount of time if the registered nurse and practical nurse work together, each respecting the other's expertise, work experience, and maturity.

If problems arise, team members should be able to discuss them intelligently and arrive at an acceptable solution. In this manner, each grows, each learns to depend on the other, and the result is a more harmonious, more efficient nursing division. It is essential to remember that one can always learn, that trust is earned, and that respect is the desire of all. One of the best ways to earn respect is to do a job well.

Student Nurse

If you are working in a hospital where there are student nurses from either the professional or the practical nursing program, remember that the objectives are the same for all—good nursing care. Ways of carrying out a procedure may vary, but the underlying principles of the procedure never change. Always use proper technique when performing any duty, procedure, or function. Proper technique is the greatest assurance of protection for the patient. In the event that you see a student or registered nurse performing a procedure that is neither correct for the patient nor in the best interest of the hospital, report this immediately to your instructor or charge nurse, who can check into the matter and make the necessary corrections.

Ancillary Personnel

To brag or boast about your accomplishments is never professional. You may be better prepared than others with whom you are working. However, this should be an incentive for you to assist your fellow workers in any way possible. Never use a condescending attitude. If a coworker has made an error and it is your responsibility to correct him, then do so in the proper manner. Call the person aside to assure privacy, and correct him in a constructive manner. If the error continues, then report the matter to the charge nurse or head nurse.

In working with nonnursing members of the health care team, always remember that these personnel have their respective supervisors who are responsible for them. Any incident or error you believe needs reporting should be reported to your charge nurse, who in turn follows the proper lines of authority to remedy the situation. Only in an emergency do you have the right to correct another hospital employee. Common sense should be used in this situation.

You win acceptance, respect, and admiration from all with whom you work by doing your job efficiently and thoroughly. This includes being cooperative, understanding, and courteous at all times.

Patient

You are an important public relations person for the hospital. The patient has so many needs to be met while he is sick that to meet these needs adequately you must acquire as much information as possible concerning his physical and mental needs. Every patient has certain capacities, interests, and desires. These are influenced by his socioeconomic background, religion, and personal and work experiences. You must know how his illness alters or affects his attitudes and behavior.

While caring for the patient's physical needs, you must recognize the emotional needs created by illness. Because humans are complex, physical and mental needs cannot be treated separately. They interact with each other; therefore they must be treated simultaneously.

Many patients find inactivity difficult. This fact is particularly true if the patient was very active before his illness. Given more time for thinking, he often develops many fears and tends to worry excessively. At times you may be able to alleviate some of these worries and fears. A simple explanation concerning procedures to be performed, an understanding attitude, and taking time to listen are some of the ways that you give the patient the assurance that he may need.

Every patient is different. Some patients may tolerate a great deal of pain, remain optimistic, and require little attention. Others, although they may experience only slight pain, may become easily depressed or require much attention from the nursing staff. The patient's forced state of helplessness may cause him to react differently from his normal state of behavior. He may hesitate to make his needs known. He may not respond to a cheerful atmosphere. He may require a serious approach. Some patients want to talk about their condition; others shy away from the subject. You must be alert to detect the patient's response and treat each patient accordingly.

You must be able to convey in some manner, either by words or actions, that you are trying to help the patient. All of your actions, the time that you spend with him, and the procedures that you must perform are done to help remedy or alleviate his present diseased condition. Unless you can convince the patient of this help, you cannot gain his cooperation, and his condition may not improve. He must have confidence in you if you are to be effective. You must have tolerance, personal self-control, and an understanding of his difficulties. Your best approach to any patient is a positive, wholesome attitude.

With a heavy work assignment and the continuing shortage of personnel in many areas, you may find it difficult to take time to listen to your patient's problems. However, allowing the patient to express his feelings may prove to be the best type of therapy. If you merely listen in a hurried manner and tell him not to worry, you have accomplished nothing for him. The patient wants to know that you understand his problems, are interested in them, and will find a solution for them if at all possible. When dealing with other people's problems, you are not emotionally involved and therefore can be more objective than they. Console the patient as much as you can in view of your understanding of his attitudes and problems.

Although a person may complain a great deal, he usually does not reveal his real worries. You should not pry into your patient's personal life, but you may ask encouraging questions that may help your patient to reveal his real problems. If you can help him to achieve a positive attitude toward solving these problems, you have given him the courage to hope again. Without hope, little can be accomplished.

Family

You must exercise tact and have a good understanding of human nature to deal with the family of your patient. The family is entrusting you, a stranger, with the care of their loved one. They want to have confidence in you, but you must instill this feeling in them.

It is difficult for the family to behave normally during the serious illness of a relative. Some families become excited and highly emotional during this time. You can alleviate some of a family's apprehension by listening to their suggestions concerning the likes and dislikes of the patient in matters of food and personal care. If these suggestions do not interfere with the physician's orders, it may prove helpful to follow them.

Any reassurance that you show to the family serves as an indirect means of helping your patient to develop a good attitude toward you and the care you are giving to him. The family and the patient must believe that you are really interested. Nursing is not just a job to be done but rather a service to be given to people.

◆ *Study Helps*

1. List the duties of a licensed practical nurse in public health. What are some of the school health services offered by the public health department?
2. What requisites are necessary for licensed practical nurses working in industry? What are their duties?
3. Explain some of the special problems encountered by a licensed practical nurse while doing private duty nursing. Who regulates salaries?
4. List the advantages available to the licensed practical nurse working in a general hospital.
5. Explain the relationship that should exist between the licensed practical nurse and the physician and the licensed practical nurse and the registered nurse.
6. What should the licensed practical nurse's attitude be toward student nurses?
7. Describe how the licensed practical nurse works effectively with ancillary personnel.
8. Explain the patient's reaction to illness. What is the responsibility of the licensed practical nurse in this area?
9. Explain the family's reaction to illness. What can the licensed practical nurse do to help them?
10. List the advantages available to the licensed practical nurse working for an agency.

Bibliography

Cookfair JM: *Nursing process and practice in the community,* St Louis, 1991, Mosby.
Deloughery G: *Issues and trends in nursing,* St Louis, 1991, Mosby.
Douglass LM: *The effective nurse,* ed 4, St Louis, 1992, Mosby.
Jaffe MS, Skidmore-Roth L: *Home health nursing care plans,* St Louis, 1988, Mosby.

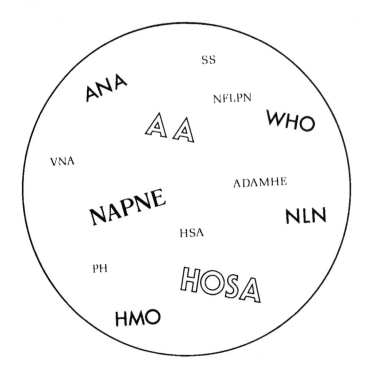

Objectives

At the completion of this chapter the student practical nurse will be able to:

♦ Explain the purposes and function of the Social Security Administration.

♦ List the functions and membership of NAPNES, NFLPN, NLN, and ANA.

♦ List five private and voluntary agencies.

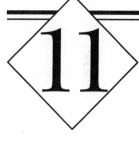

11 Organizations, Insurance, and Agencies

◆ Nursing Organizations

National Association for Practical Nurse Education and Service (NAPNES)

NAPNES (1400 Spring Street, Suite 310, Silver Spring, MD 20910), established in 1941, was the first organization for promoting schools of practical nursing and the welfare and continuing education of licensed practical nurses.

In 1959 a new department, the Department of Service to State Practical Nurse Associations, was added. It assists state organizations of practical nursing with any operational and educational problems.

Membership in this organization includes practical nurses, practical nursing students, directors and instructors of schools of practical nursing, nursing home administrators, physicians, professional nurses, and interested lay persons. Membership fees are paid annually either as individual members or through membership in the state association. The subscription to the association's official magazine, the *Journal of Practical Nursing*, is included in the fee. Some of the functions of this organization are as follows:

1. Providing educational material for faculties to use in practical nursing
2. Providing a current list of approved schools of practical nursing throughout the country
3. Providing resource personnel for workshops, state conferences, and summer courses for practical nursing educators
4. Recruiting practical nursing students by publicizing and distributing information about practical nursing
5. Collaborating with other nursing organizations in the health field
6. Providing ways for licensed practical nurses to continue their education by sponsoring workshops and encouraging the development and accreditation of postlicensure programs
7. Providing for the welfare of the licensed practical nurse by publishing informa-

tion about legal aspects of practical nursing, keeping the licensed practical nurse informed about legislation, and sponsoring low-cost group insurance programs

8. Publishing the *Journal of Practical Nursing*

The voting body, which is made up of the constituent state associations, determines the broad policies of the association. The general management responsibility of the association rests with the board of directors; the majority of the members are licensed practical nurses. Standing committees are assigned many of the activities of the association. These standing committees sometimes delegate tasks to work committees. Provision is made in the bylaws for the formation of councils. Council members are in groups that have special interests in common.

National Federation of Licensed Practical Nurses, Inc. (NFLPN)

NFLPN (3948 Browning Place, PO Box 18088, Raleigh, NC 27619) is the national membership organization and is the policy-making body for licensed practical nurses. NFLPN is the only organization that is composed entirely of licensed practical nurses and serves constituent state associations of like structure. The organization was formed in 1949 by a group of licensed practical nurses to gain status and recognition and to provide an official channel through which licensed practical nurses could speak, act, and work independently on their own behalf.

Members in this organization are licensed practical nurses and student practical nurses, who may participate in some of the local and state activities. Membership dues are paid once a year; a certain portion of the dues is set aside for national membership dues and the official magazine *The Journal of Nursing Care*. NFLPN has two types of members. The first are members who join NFLPN through the constituent state association or as members-at-large. The latter members are those who live in a state that is not a constituent member of NFLPN.

Some functions of this organization are as follows:

1. Providing an accrediting program for schools that want to be accredited as having met the required standards formulated by NFPLN.
2. Concerning itself with the principles of ethics and continuing education for the licensed practical nurse to improve patient care
3. Keeping its members informed concerning matters of interest through the use of letters, bulletins, and appropriate speakers to improve practice
4. Making available to its members health, malpractice, accident, and personal liability insurance plans
5. Working with legislation as the spokesperson on the national level for important matters pertaining to practical nursing
6. Cooperating with other organizations in the health field in the interest of quality and total patient care
7. Continuing to work for licensed practical nurse representation on state boards of nursing
8. Providing a statement of functions and qualifications of the licensed practical nurse that reflects the expanding role of the practical nurse
9. Encouraging all employing agencies to provide in-service education
10. Striving to improve leadership within the organization

In 1972 the NFLPN's House of Delegates passed some major resolutions in the areas of continuing education, standards of licensure, and nursing practice acts. They recommended the study of the concept of mandatory continuing education as a requirement for renewal of a license until such time as an effective method of administration is developed. They recommended that NFLPN go on record as approving the National League for Nursing State Board Test Pool Examination as the standard for licensure. They also recommended that NFLPN support the updating of nursing practice acts to identify licensed practical nurses as peer participants on the professional team responsible for health care delivery and to include the NFLPN definition of practical nursing.

The licensed practical nurse is prepared to function as a member of the health care team by exercising sound nursing judgment based on preparation, knowledge, skills, understanding, and past experiences in nursing situations. But the NFLPN's recommendations show that the practical nurse must keep up with rapid changes to meet the increasing responsibilities.

National League for Nursing, Inc. (NLN)

In 1952 the NLN (350 Hudson Street, New York, NY 10014 with branch offices in San Francisco and Atlanta) was established by combining programs and resources of three national organizations and four committees. These were the National League for Nursing Education, the Association of Collegiate Schools of Nursing, the National Organization for Public Health Nursing, the Joint Committee on Practical Nurses and Auxiliary Workers in Nursing, the National Committee for the Improvement of Nursing Services, the National Accrediting Service, and the Joint Committee on Careers in Nursing.

NLN membership includes individual members and agency members. An individual member is any person interested in health care and nursing from throughout the United States. Agency members are nursing schools and nursing services.

The NLN has numerous functions that help the nursing profession. It has a department for professional and practical nursing programs. Some functions of this department include the following:

1. Preparing the examination for licensure given to nursing students
2. Accrediting schools of nursing
3. Issuing a current list of scholarships, education grants, and loans for continuing education in the nursing field
4. Informing its members about current issues under evaluation and those newly formulated
5. Cooperating with legislation on the national level in important matters pertaining to nursing
6. Publishing a monthly newsletter that is distributed to all individual and agency members
7. Providing consultation and assistance to programs of nursing as needed
8. Conducting workshops for instructors of schools of nursing throughout the country and providing resource personnel
9. Providing a current list of approved schools of nursing throughout the country
10. Issuing guides to those desiring to establish schools of nursing
11. Providing educational material for use in nursing
12. Publishing *Nursing and Health Care*

The organization is strictly a nursing organization and strives to improve all phases and levels of nursing and nursing care.

NLN Council of Practical Nursing Programs

In 1957 the Council of Practical Nursing Programs was founded. It is concerned with development and improvement of educational programs in practical nursing. The Board of Review for Practical Nursing Programs is appointed by the executive committee and is responsible for evaluating NLN accreditation of practical nursing education. Agency members work together to raise standards and to improve practical nurse preparation within the programs. The Council of Practical Nursing Programs recognizes the need and urges licensed practical nurses to increase their education by taking educational courses that are available.

American Nurses' Association (ANA)

The national organization and official representative for all professional registered nurses is the ANA (2420 Pershing Road, Kansas City, MO 64108), founded in 1896. The ANA is to the professional registered nurse what the NFLPN is to the licensed practical nurse. The members of this organization are kept informed through its official publications, the *American Journal of Nursing* and *The American Nurse*. The ANA is like the previously discussed nursing organizations in that it works closely with other health and welfare organizations.

Health Occupations Students of America (HOSA)

In 1976, HOSA (New Jersey Department of Education, Division of Vocational Education, 225 West State Street, Trenton, NJ 08625) was founded as a national vocational organization. State and local chapters provide activities and programs to help students in health occupations develop their mental, social, and physical well-being. Interactions with student organizations, businesses, and professions strengthen members in leadership and citizenship abilities, in appreciation of helping people, and in developing good decision-making skills. As a practical nursing student, you have the opportunity to meet students in other health careers and to improve health conditions in the community through this organization. For information pertaining to state and local chapters contact your state department of education or vocational technical education.

Your Alumni Organization

On completion of your program of practical nursing in your respective school, you should want to join your alumni organization. This gives you a feeling of being united with your classmates and other graduates from your school. By attending alumni meetings you keep up with the progress that your school is making. Often you can help to better the educational program of your school through constructive suggestions. It also gives you an opportunity to familiarize yourself with new developments that are taking place in a hospital as related by an alumnus working in that particular institution. Because membership means "belonging," you have the obligation to be an active member if you join your alumni organization. Plans for continuing education programs are often provided through alumni activities. Projects may be established to provide funds for scholarships to be used by future students in your school. Your alumni organization seeks to encourage the present students to achieve their goals. This may be in the form of an annual tea for the students, a banquet, or a program of entertainment for the students and their parents. Annual dues may be used to enroll officers annually in the national practical nursing organizations or to meet the ever constant need for educational equipment for your school. Your school provided you with the type of education you were seeking; now you should be willing to help other needy students in the school as well as the school itself.

◆ Health and Welfare Insurance, Organizations, and Agencies

Health Insurance

Many types of insurance are available in the United States to protect individuals from some of the financial costs of accidents and illnesses.

Medicare, the health insurance plan under the Social Security Act, went into effect July 1, 1966. Under this plan basic hospital benefits and voluntary supplementary medical insurance were made available for 19 million citizens 65 years of age and older. Since 1966 new Social Security legislation has been enacted, and the benefits of the program have expanded. Some states offer other programs in conjunction with the federal government to help defray medical expenses for low income residents or welfare assistance recipients. This program is known as Medicaid; eligibility and requirements vary in different states.

Medicare includes two parts. Part A is the hospital insurance and is financed by special contributions from employers, employees, and self-employed persons. Part B is the medical insurance; it is financed jointly by the federal government and by the basic medical insurance policies of those who enroll voluntarily when they become 65 years of age.

Part A (hospital insurance) helps to pay some hospitalization costs and contributes to related health services that may be required when the patient leaves the hospital. The hospital benefits are limited to certain maximum amounts for specified periods of time. The "benefit period" may begin again if the person has not received skilled nursing care for 60 consecutive days. Some benefits included are as follows:

1. Inpatient hospital benefits include semiprivate rooms with regular nursing care; meals, including special diets; operating room charges, including recovery room charges; intensive care nursing; medical supplies such as traction, braces, crutches, and walkers; social services; drugs; laboratory tests; and x-ray examinations and other radiology services.

2. Extended care benefits after leaving the hospital, provided the physician determines the patient needs such care, are the same as the hospital benefits shown previously. The physician must order care in an extended care facility (ECF) at least 3 days after hospitalization or within 14 days after the patient has left the hospital.

3. Home health benefits are available when the physician decides that continued care is needed in the patient's home by a home health agency following the patient's discharge from a hospital or ECF. These benefits include social ser-

vices; speech, occupational, and physical therapy; part-time nursing and home health aide care; and the use of medical supplies and medical appliances.

Part B (medical insurance) helps pay for some of the patient's covered medical expenses when they exceed the specified amount that is deductible each year. Some benefits included are as follows:

1. Physician's service in the office, in the outpatient department, at home, or in the hospital
2. Drugs that must be administered by the physician and cannot be self-administered
3. Hospital outpatient services, including diagnosis and treatment (special limitations on psychiatric care)
4. Specified services of a podiatrist
5. Miscellaneous health and medical services ordered by a physician, such as diagnostic services; x-ray and radiation treatments; physical therapy; surgical dressings, casts, and braces; and rental of equipment such as a hospital bed, walker, or other equipment to be used in the home

Of the approximately 2000 private insurance agencies, Blue Cross is the largest single supplier of hospital insurance. Its plans usually cover the hospital room, regular nursing care, laboratory services, x-ray examinations, electrocardiograms, drugs, dressings, special treatments, operating and delivery rooms, and many other hospital services. Membership must be transferred when members move to another area. Hospitalization insurance should be included in the family budget because hospital care is a part of life.

Various types of insurance plans are designed to help meet the costs of sickness and accidents. Blue Cross and Blue Shield policies are generally accepted as the main plans in many areas of the country. Many plans encourage the use of preventive care (health maintenance organizations) and cover medical costs for the insured even when there is no hospitalization. You should know and understand the policy before you take it, because the benefits, including length of time covered, surgery, medical expenses, and nursing care, may vary greatly with each policy.

For several years now much has been said about the need for an effective form of national health insurance to benefit all citizens. Several plans have been proposed, but there seems to be no real agreement at this time as to which kind of plan is needed.

Some type of plan that offers unlimited possibilities for new kinds of health care undoubtedly will be developed within the coming years. Be sure to follow political developments and proposals closely through nursing journals and other sources. It is possible that you, the practical nurse, will be involved in the planning stages of preventive care and health education.

Health Maintenance Organization (HMO)

A health maintenance organization is a prepaid, highly organized system of health care. The concept of the HMO is aimed at preventing illness and maintaining health through routine health examinations, close observation, early diagnosis of disease, and health teaching. Members of an HMO pay a monthly or quarterly membership fee and for this receive standard, essential health services.

The prevention of disease is a medically and economically sound philosophy. It costs less to keep persons healthy than to cure them once they are ill. A diagnostic office visit is cheaper than a stay in the hospital.

Once a client becomes a member of an HMO he is entitled to all the services. He must choose as his primary physician one of the HMO's staff. The physician employed by the HMO receives a salary, and this salary is not based on the number of patients he sees. A member's fee, too, remains the same whether he sees a physician once a year or once a week. All basic health services are rendered at a central location. Some large HMOs have their own hospitals; however, most have contracts with hospitals that provide many varied and diagnostic services.

Nurses are an important part of an HMO. They function as primary health practitioners, working with physicians, not for physicians.

Government Health and Welfare Organizations

To provide better care for the patient in the community and to promote health and the prevention of illness, hospitals are now working closely with many health and welfare organizations outside the hospital.

Department of Health and Human Services (DHHS). The DHHS, established in 1953 as the Department of Health, Education, and Welfare, helps promote the general welfare of the entire population. It has been reorganized several times to better meet its many responsibilities. To carry out fully its programs in health, welfare, vocational rehabilitation, consumer protection, and social security, Title VI of the Civil Rights Act of 1964 prohibiting discrimination needed to be enforced. Major reorganizations again occurred in 1966 after the creation of a new administration on aging. The largest amount of money is used by nonfederal agencies, institutions, and individuals necessitating various partnerships for the improvement of our society.

The DDHS is a cabinet-level department, with the Secretary advising the President on programs of the federal government pertaining to welfare, health, and income security plans. The DHHS is concerned with people of all ages, from newborn infants to the elderly, by mailing out social security checks and making health services more widely available.

Office of Human Development Services (OHDS). The OHDS administers programs designed to deal with specific population problems, such as children of low income families, handicapped persons, runaway youth, the elderly, native Americans, native Alaskans, and native Hawaiians (see Fig. 11-1).

Social Security Administration. The Social Security Administration was established in 1935 by the U.S. government. As the needs of the people changed, the basic program has been changed. This national health program includes old age, survivors', and disability insurance, which now covers almost all persons who are employed (see Fig. 11-1).

Most working persons in the United States are now establishing protection for themselves and their families by paying their Social Security contributions. During working years, employees, their employers, and self-employed people pay social security contributions into a special trust fund. When a worker retires, becomes disabled, or

OFFICE OF HUMAN DEVELOPMENT SERVICES

Administration for:

Aging

Children, Youth, and Families

Native Americans

Developmental Disabilities

Office of Policy, Planning, and Legislation

PUBLIC HEALTH SERVICES

Centers for Disease Control

Food and Drug Administration

Health Resources and Services Administration

National Institutes of Health

Alcohol, Drug Abuse, and Mental Health Administration

Agency for Toxic Substances and Disease Registry

HEALTH CARE FINANCING ADMINISTRATION

Office of Executive Operations

Office of the Associate Administrator for:

External Affairs

Management and Support Services

Operations

Program Development

SOCIAL SECURITY ADMINISTRATION

Office of:

System Operations

Hearings and Appeals

Disability

Assessment

Management, Budget, and Personnel

The Actuary

Central Operations

Policy

FAMILY SUPPORT ADMINISTRATION

Office of:

Family Assistance

Refugee Resettlement

Child Support Enforcement

Community Services

Fig. 11-1 Federal health and welfare organizations. Modified from Department of Health & Human Services.

dies, benefits in the form of monthly checks are paid to individuals or families to replace part of the earnings lost. Part of the contributions go into a hospital trust fund that is used to help pay hospital bills when workers and their dependents reach 65. Because changes occur rapidly, contact the Social Security office nearest you for current information.

Administered by each state, social security insurance against other risks is provided through workmen's compensation and unemployment insurance. In addition to these social security insurance programs, a program of federal grants to the states helps provide financial assistance, medical care, and other services for each state's needy people.

Social Security cards. Nursing is covered by the Social Security Act; thus you must have a Social Security number. This number, which is shown on your Social Security card, is used to keep a record of your earnings. You should use the same number all your life. Both your name and number are needed to make sure that you get credit for your earnings. You should show your card to each employer so that your name and number are used to report your wages correctly. If you are self-employed, copy your name and number exactly as they appear on the card on the form you use to report your net earnings for Social Security credit.

If a Social Security office is in your town, you may get a Social Security card or get a duplicate card to replace one if it is lost or if you change your name. Be sure the new card shows the same number. If no Social Security office is in your town, you may obtain an application blank from your post office.

The law requires each employer to give you a receipt for the Social Security taxes that have been deducted from your pay. This is done at the end of each year and when you terminate employment. These receipts (W-2 forms) help you check on your Social Security because they show the amount deducted as well as the wages paid you. You may check the total earnings reported for you by obtaining an addressed postcard from your Social Security office, signing it, and sending it back, or you may write the Social Security Administration, Baltimore, MD 21235, and request a statement of your account. This statement shows the amount of earnings reported for you. It does not show the amount of taxes paid. Benefits are based on earnings, not on the amount of taxes paid.

Public Health Service. The Public Health Service (Room 17-22, 5600 Fishers Lane, Rockville, MD 20852), created by an act in 1789, has been broadened to cover the responsibility of improving and protecting the environment and health of the people of the nation. This service also works in cooperation with other countries and international organizations involved in world health care planning. Since 1967 the Public Health Service has been divided into six major agencies: Centers for Disease Control; Food and Drug Administration; Health Resources and Services Administration; National Institutes of Health; Alcohol, Drug Abuse, and Mental Health Administration; and Agency for Toxic Substances and Disease Registry.

Food and Drug Administration. The Food and Drug Administration (HFI-10, 5600 Fishers Lane, Rockville, MD 20852) was established in 1906 and has been known under several organizational titles. It is made up of several bureaus the main functions of which are to protect the health of the nation against potential hazards, impure and unsafe drugs, foods, and cosmetics. Some examples are (1) research programs conducted to study biological effects and long-term exposure to potentially toxic chemicals; (2) policies on labeling all drugs, evaluation of new drugs, quality of drugs, and effectiveness of over-the-counter drugs; and (3) standards set up after research on food for quality, safety, food additives, nutrition, and cosmetics.

National Institutes of Health. The National Institutes of Health (Building #1, Room 307, Bethesda, MD 20014) was established to improve the American people's health. This is accomplished by conducting research into the causes, prevention, and cure of disease; developing and supporting research training and services; and communicating biological and medical information using current methods.

This organization is made up of several institutes and divisions for specific subjects, such as the National Institute on Aging.

Alcohol, Drug Abuse, and Mental Health Administration. This administration (Room 16-95, 5600 Fishers Lane, Rockville, MD 20852) was established at the federal level to provide leadership in the reduction and elimination of alcohol and drug abuse health problems. This organization is responsible for prevention, control, treatment, and rehabilitation of persons affected by alcohol abuse, drug abuse, and mental illness.

Health Services Administration. The Health Services Administration (Room 14A-55, 5600 Fishers Lane, Rockville, MD 20852) was established to provide leadership in the delivery of health services. Through bureaus, health care services are provided for migrant workers, maternal and child welfare, family planning, community health, native Americans, federal beneficiaries, and native Alaskans. These services are provided through hospitals, clinics, and ambulatory health care centers in urban and rural areas.

Food stamp program. The food stamp program was initiated in 1961 by the Department of Agriculture as a method for helping low income and welfare-aided families to buy needed food. The federal government makes up the difference between the amount the family pays and the total value of the coupons. The coupons may be used to buy all foods, excluding those imported.

State health departments. State health departments are supported by state funds and are under the jurisdiction of the governors of the states, who appoint various officials responsible for the local departments. The departments and officials included vary from state to state. Some state health departments are responsible for the licensing of nursing homes, hospitals, undertakers, beauticians, and manufacturers, as well as for providing film libraries, assistance to the local departments, and educational materials (usually free). Other state divisions work in the areas of mental health, nutrition, venereal disease, vital statistics, communicable disease control, public health nursing, laboratories, research, sanitation, and maternal and child health.

Local health departments. Local health departments have many of the same duties as the state health departments; however, the functions differ with each county, city, or township, depending on available funds and their use. The quality and quantity of services given are affected at the local level by the mayor, county supervisor, councilpersons, county managers, and commissioners. Their routine responsibilities ordinarily include (1) reporting all communicable diseases; (2) maternal and child health, dental health, nutrition, mental health, and schools; (3) vital statistics and accurate record keeping of birth, death, population, disease, marriage, and divorce rates; (4) environmental sanitation; and (5) public health nursing and health education.

World Health Organization (WHO). The main function of WHO is to assist countries in strengthening their own health services through the advice of public health experts in disease control. Other functions include international sanitary regulations, uniform registration of diseases and deaths, standardization of important drugs, and control of communicable diseases throughout the world.

Private and Voluntary Health Agencies

Private and voluntary health agencies receive funds through donations, gifts, United Way, membership fees, and sometimes public funds. Public funds may be given to a voluntary hospital as payment for some service that is considered a public responsibility, such as for an indigent patient.

Because of difficulties incurred through administration at a national level, most private agencies are operated on a state or local level. If you have no agency in your area to meet a specific need and help is needed for your patient, you may write to the National Health Council, 1740 Broadway, New York, NY 10019, for the location of the nearest state or local office.

Some of these private and voluntary agencies are as follows:

1. *Alcoholics Anonymous*—helps any alcoholic who desires help. Alcoholics Anonymous groups throughout the world are made up of recovered alcoholics. They share their recovery to help other alcoholics overcome their problem.
2. *American Cancer Society*—constitutes a threefold program of research, education, and service aimed at controlling and eliminating cancer. It provides service and rehabilitation counseling, transportation, and loan-closet items (sickroom supplies and comfort items). Volunteers assist in rehabilitation of laryngectomy, mastectomy, and ostomy patients. Other patient assistance programs specific to each local division are also available.
3. *American Diabetes Association*—provides education to the public and to professionals regarding the nature and treatment of diabetes. It distributes accurate information to the public and to patients. It improves standards of treatment and promotes research.
4. *American Heart Association, Inc.*—provides educational programs for professionals, patients, and the general public. It supports research and sets standards to maintain better medical care for patients with cardiovascular diseases.
5. *American National Red Cross*—was chosen by the Congress to help carry out the obligations assumed by the United States under certain international treaties

known as the Geneva or Red Cross Conventions. A volunteer 50-member board of governors directs the activities of the Red Cross, which are carried out by the managers of four national field offices through 70 divisions and 3142 local chapters. The congressional charter imposes on the American Red Cross two of its programs: services to the armed forces, veterans, and their families and disaster services. Other programs, all of which are designed to meet human needs, are the blood program, community health and safety programs (first aid, small craft, water safety, and nursing and health), youth service programs, community volunteer programs, and international services.

6. *Arthritis and Rheumatism Foundation*—conducts research, promotes educational programs, supports treatment facilities, and assists in training physicians and other health care personnel in prevention, diagnosis, and treatment of arthritis.

7. *Association for the Aid of Crippled Children* (and adults)—offers instructional materials, conducts research and scientific conferences for health care providers, and prepares educational literature for patients. This organization receives some funds from Easter Seals.

8. *Muscular Dystrophy Association of America, Inc.*—conducts research for the discovery of a cause and cure for muscular dystrophy. It assists in the purchase and repair of appliances and provides physical therapy, transportation, education, and counseling.

9. *National Society for the Prevention of Blindness*—cooperates with local organizations such as parents' groups, fraternal organizations, health-related institutions, and governmental agencies in sight conservation programs. It gives vision-screening tests and publishes a wide variety of educational and teaching materials. It offers industry safety incentive programs and awards research grants in a wide variety of areas with potential application to prevention of blindness.

10. *National Association for Mental Health*—conducts clinical research, provides educational programs, and works for improved preventive and treatment facilities. It informs the public about ways to avoid mental breakdown.

11. *National Coordinating Council of Drug Abuse*—evaluates educational programs, assists in research, and sets up interdisciplinary committees by area needs. It coordinates educational and informational efforts of groups on drug abuse.

12. *National Multiple Sclerosis Society*—offers a research program in finding the cause, treatment, and cure of this disease. It provides educational literature for health care providers, victims, and the public.

13. *Planned Parenthood*—conducts research, makes educational literature available, and deals with issues of family size, child spacing, marriage, infertility, and family stability.

14. *Visiting Nurses' Association*—provides nursing at home under a physician's orders for the acutely ill, chronically ill, invalids, mothers and newborn babies, convalescents, and others who are unable to leave home for treatment. This agency teaches members of the family to give patient care, as well as assisting the patient in regaining and maintaining health.

In addition to the organizations listed, many programs are administered at the local level.

◆ Home Care-Related Organizations

The following is a partial list of the national groups and associations that may help the home care giver.

Aging

American Association of Retired Persons (AARP)
1909 K St., N.W.
Washington, DC 20049
(202) 872-4700
The National Association of Area Agencies on Aging (N4A)
600 Maryland Ave., S.W.
Suite 208-W
Washington, DC 20024
(202) 484-7520
National Support Center for Families of the Aging
P.O. Box 245
Swarthmore, PA 19081

Home Care

Foundation for Hospice and Homecare
519 C St., N.E.
Stanton Park
Washington, DC 20002
(202) 547-6586
National Association for Home Care
519 C St., N.E.
Stanton Park
Washington, DC 20002
(202) 547-7424

Self-Help Clearing Houses

The National Self Help Clearinghouse
c/o City University of New York
33 W. 42nd St.
New York, NY 10036
(212) 840-1259
The Self Help Center
1600 Dodge Ave.
Suite S-122
Evanston, IL 60201
(312) 328-0470

◆ *Study Helps*

1. List two journals published especially for the practical nurse and give the publisher of each.
2. Explain NAPNES and state its functions.
3. Explain NFLPN and state its functions.
4. Explain NLN and state its functions.
5. Explain ANA and state its functions.
6. What is the purpose of an alumni organization? What is your obligation toward it?
7. List six health and welfare organizations and state their functions.

Bibliography

Cornacchia HJ, Barrett S: *Consumer health: a guide to intelligent decisions,* ed 5, St Louis, 1992, Mosby.
De Young L: *Dynamics of nursing,* ed 5, St Louis, 1984, Mosby.
Ebersole P, Hess P: *Toward healthy aging,* ed 3, St Louis, 1994, Mosby.
Reinhardt AM, Quinn MD: *Family-centered community nursing,* St Louis, 1980, Mosby.
Saxton DF, Nugent PM, Pelikan PK: *Mosby's comprehensive review of nursing,* ed 13, St Louis, 1990, Mosby.

APPENDIX A

Desirable Characteristics for a Leader

1. Listens and is approachable
2. Communicates clearly verbally and in writing
3. Sets high standards; is honest and trustworthy
4. Is fair and objective
5. Is a doer and sets a positive example
6. Uses positive motivational techniques
7. Is goal-oriented and organized
8. Shows enthusiasm and a sense of humor
9. Is tactful, humble, and understanding
10. Is knowledgeable and has good judgment

APPENDIX B   Styles of Leadership

Those of you with work experience have probably seen several leadership styles in action. Those of you who have not held jobs can think of teachers or head nurses in clinical agencies that you visited during school.

None of the styles discussed in this appendix is right or wrong. The most effective leaders frequently use more than one style. The art of leadership is knowing which style to use at a given time. Much may be learned by observing people in leadership roles and comparing them to the descriptions given below.

◆ Authoritarian Style

Some individuals feel that because they have authority or power they should "call the shots" on everything. They often tend to be poor communicators and like to "tell" everybody under their direction what, when, and how to do everything. They let you know immediately that they are the boss. The technical name for this style of leadership is the authoritarian or autocratic style. Authoritarian leaders often do not trust others. They frequently believe that people do not want to work and will do anything to get out of working. Because of this distrust they feel a strong need to maintain control. Most people do not like to work for highly authoritarian leaders, because this style does not allow individual employees to contribute or participate actively in work-related decisions. Most people are likely to be afraid of authoritarian leaders because they have a tendency to be highly critical.

Newly appointed supervisors or team leaders frequently act in an authoritarian manner. This happens for several reasons. Some training programs tend to be authoritarian. The student is expected to follow instructions and not question directions. It is natural for students to model their behaviors on familiar ideas, even if they know that they are not the most effective actions.

Fear may also be a factor when adopting the authoritarian style. When persons are uncertain but wish to appear in control, it is easier to give orders that seem to indicate knowledge and confidence than to acknowledge that an assistant may have valuable knowledge to contribute. Frequently student nurses are expected to have the right answer when questioned by the instructor; indications of uncertainty are not acceptable.

This thinking carries over into the new situation and makes admission of the need for help awkward.

Lack of trust is another reason new supervisors adopt the authoritarian style. When they begin to supervise, they realize that they are accepting responsibility for the actions of other people. This comes as a shock to many new supervisors. They have often just gained enough confidence to trust themselves. Suddenly they have to make the additional mental shift to trusting others. This is difficult, particularly for new graduates. Many people feel that if they give orders and exercise a great deal of control, everything will run smoothly.

Poor communication skills may also be a factor in the authoritarian style. Persons who have poor communication skills may have to resort to giving orders. They lack many of the techniques that allow them to do anything else.

Do not infer from this discussion that the authoritarian style is without merit. There are times when giving directions or orders is not only proper, it is necessary.

◆ Democratic Style

Another style of leadership that you may have observed is the democratic style. This is also called the collaborative or participative style of leadership. Democratic leaders are in charge. They are responsible for providing direction to the group. The difference between authoritarian and democratic styles is that the participative leaders attempt to include all of the staff in the decision-making process. Group members are actively involved in setting goals; therefore they are usually more committed to seeing that these goals are achieved.

Democratic leaders usually have a view of others different from that of authoritarian leaders. They are more likely to trust others, usually because they have greater confidence themselves. They think that others want to work and desire to do their jobs well. Good understanding of communications and human relations skills is a common trait of democratic leaders. Authoritarian leaders gives orders, whereas democratic leaders guide and direct. In most cases groups working under democratic leaders get more work done and are happier doing the work.

There is also a negative side to the democratic style. Establishing a democratic climate takes time. It takes a group of strangers time to learn to trust democratic leaders. Because this style is not familiar to many people, they may not be sure whether the leader really wants their input. It also takes longer to get ideas and information from several people before making a decision than it takes if one person makes the decision.

◆ Laissez-Faire Style

This term comes from the French language. The literal translation is "allow them to do." Another way of saying this is "anything goes." Laissez-faire leaders do not interfere but let others do as they please. Some individuals who have grown up in a very authoritarian system go to the opposite extreme and never give orders or directions. This frequently results in chaos, with little work being accomplished. Because there is no direction or guidance in a laissez-faire system, persons often are confused and unsure of what is expected of them. This is not an effective style in most settings, and in a health care setting it may result in total disaster.

◆ Task-Oriented Style Versus People-Oriented Style

Some supervisors focus on accomplishing tasks. They see a day as a list of jobs to be done. This list of tasks is divided among the staff until everything gets done. Little attention is paid to the people who have to do the work. The workers are viewed as a means to an end. Individual abilities, likes, and dislikes are all secondary to getting the job done. Most nurses tend to be task-oriented. They frequently see their day as a list of orders, medications, appointments, and treatments. This is an unrealistic perception of the profession. Because of this approach they may lose track of others, both patients and employees. People-oriented leaders focus more on the individual involved than the tasks. They may know that the tasks are important, but they do not want to hurt anybody's feelings. However, this situation rarely lasts because the tasks are not completed as expected.

The most workable style is a combination of the task-oriented and people-oriented styles. The ideal is to balance the task- and people-oriented attitude. This combination recognizes that many tasks are to be done, but that the people involved are important also.

◆ Situational or Eclectic Style

As stated earlier no single style is always appropriate. The most effective leaders select aspects from several styles as the situation requires. Eclectic leaders realize that both the tasks and the persons involved are important. In situations involving nursing care the supervising nurse must keep complete control. If something must be done, or must be done in a particular way, it is the leader's responsibility to see that it is done promptly and correctly. Nurses reporting to the supervisor must recognize her authority and responsibility. In cases of emergency the supervisor must know that an order will be followed.

In other areas, however, the nurse in charge may use a more democratic style. Making daily assignments, assigning miscellaneous tasks, and scheduling breaks and lunch are simple examples of where the employees could and should have input. These areas affect the employee directly and greatly affect job satisfaction.

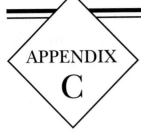

Leadership and Followership Style Test

◆ Structural Leadership Profile

The following 20 statements relate to your ideal image of leadership. We ask that as you respond to them, you imagine yourself to be a leader and then answer the questions in a way that would reflect your particular style of leadership. It makes no difference what kind of leadership experience, if any, you have had or are currently involved in. The purpose here is to establish your ideal preference for relating with subordinates.

The format includes a 5-point scale ranging from *strongly agree* to *strongly disagree* for each statement. Please select one point on each scale and mark it as you read the 20 statements relating to leadership. You may omit answers to questions that are confusing or to questions that you feel you cannot answer.

	STRONGLY AGREE	AGREE	MIXED FEELINGS	DISAGREE	STRONGLY DISAGREE
1. When I tell a subordinate to do something I expect him/her to do it with no questions asked. After all, I am responsible for what he/she will do, not the subordinate.	1	2	3	4	5
2. Tight control by a leader usually does more harm than good. People will generally do the best job when they are allowed to exercise self-control.	5	4	3	2	1
3. Although discipline is important in an organization, the effective leader should mediate the use of disciplinary procedures with his/her knowledge of the people and the situation.	1	2	3	4	5

Continued

Leadership and Followership Style Test—continued

	STRONGLY AGREE	AGREE	MIXED FEELINGS	DISAGREE	STRONGLY DISAGREE
4. A leader must make every effort to subdivide the tasks of the people to the greatest possible extent.	1	2	3	4	5
5. Shared leadership or truly democratic process in a group can only work when there is a recognized leader who assists the process.	1	2	3	4	5
6. As a leader I am ultimately responsible for all of the actions of my group. If our activities result in benefits for the organization I should be rewarded accordingly.	1	2	3	4	5
7. Most persons require only minimum direction on the part of their leader in order to do a good job.	5	4	3	2	1
8. One's subordinates usually require the control of a strict leader.	1	2	3	4	5
9. Leadership might be shared among participants of a group so that at any one time there could be two or more leaders.	5	4	3	2	1
10. Leadership should generally come from the top, but there are some logical exceptions to this rule.	5	4	3	2	1
11. The disciplinary function of the leader is simply to seek democratic opinions regarding problems as they arise.	5	4	3	2	1
12. The engineering problems, the management time, and the worker frustration caused by the division of labor are hardly ever worth the savings. In most cases, workers could do the best job of determining their own job content.	5	4	3	2	1
13. The leader ought to be the group member whom the other members elect to coordinate their activities and to represent the group to the rest of the organization.	5	4	3	2	1
14. A leader needs to exercise some control over his/her people.	1	2	3	4	5
15. There must be one and only one recognized leader in a group.	1	2	3	4	5

Leadership and Followership Style Test—continued

	STRONGLY AGREE	AGREE	MIXED FEELINGS	DISAGREE	STRONGLY DISAGREE
16. A good leader must establish and strictly enforce an impersonal system of discipline.	1	2	3	4	5
17. Discipline codes should be flexible and they should allow for individual decisions by the leader, given each particular situation.	5	4	3	2	1
18. Basically, people are responsible for themselves and no one else. Thus a leader cannot be blamed for or take credit for the work of subordinates.	5	4	3	2	1
19. The job of the leader is to relate to subordinates the task to be done, to ask them for the ways in which it can best be accomplished, and then to help arrive at a consensus plan of attack.	5	4	3	2	1
20. A position of leadership implies the general superiority of its incumbent over his/her workers.	1	2	3	4	5

◆ Structural Followership Profile

This section of the questionnaire includes statements about the type of boss you prefer. Imagine yourself to be in a subordinate position of some kind and use your responses to indicate your preference for the way in which a leader might relate with you. The format will be identical to that within the previous section.

1. I expect my job to be very explicitly outlined for me.	1	2	3	4	5
2. When the boss says to do something, I do it. After all, he/she is the boss.	1	2	3	4	5
3. Rigid rules and regulations usually cause me to become frustrated and inefficient.	5	4	3	2	1
4. I am ultimately responsible for and capable of self-discipline based upon my contacts with the people around me.	5	4	3	2	1
5. My jobs should be made as short in duration as possible, so that I can achieve efficiency through repetition.	1	2	3	4	5

Continued

Leadership and Followership Style Test—continued

	STRONGLY AGREE	AGREE	MIXED FEELINGS	DISAGREE	STRONGLY DISAGREE
6. Within reasonable limits I will try to accommodate requests from persons who are not my boss since these requests are typically in the best interest of the company anyhow.	5	4	3	2	1
7. When the boss tells me to do something which is the wrong thing to do, it is his/her fault, not mine when I do it.	1	2	3	4	5
8. It is up to my leader to provide a set of rules by which I can measure my performance.	1	2	3	4	5
9. The boss is the boss. And the fact of that promotion suggests that he/she has something on the ball.	1	2	3	4	5
10. I only accept orders from my boss.	1	2	3	4	5
11. I would prefer for my boss to give me general objectives and guidelines and then allow me to do the job my way.	5	4	3	2	1
12. If I do something which is not right it is my own fault, even if my supervisor told me to do it.	5	4	3	2	1
13. I prefer jobs which are not repetitious, the kind of task which is new and different each time.	5	4	3	2	1
14. My supervisor is in no way superior to me by virtue of position. He/she does a different kind of job, one which includes a lot of managing and coordinating.	5	4	3	2	1
15. I expect my leader to give me disciplinary guidelines.	1	2	3	4	5
16. I prefer to tell my supervisor what I will or at least should be doing. It is I who is ultimately responsible for my own work.	5	4	3	2	1

◆ Scoring Interpretation

You may score your own leadership and followership styles by simply averaging the numbers below your answers to the individual items. For example, if you scored item number one *strongly agree* you will find the point value of "1" below that answer (Leadership Profile). To obtain your overall leadership style add all the numerical values which are associated with the 20 leadership items and divide by 20. The resulting average is your leadership style.

◆ Interpretations

SCORE	DESCRIPTION	LEADERSHIP STYLE	FOLLOWERSHIP STYLE
Less than 1.9	Very autocratic	Boss decides and announces decisions, rules, orientation	Can't function well without programs and procedures. Needs feedback.
2.0–2.4	Moderately autocratic	Announces decisions but asks for questions, makes exceptions to rules	Needs solid structure and feedback but can also carry on independently
2.5–3.4	Mixed	Boss suggests ideas and consults groups, many exceptions to regulations	Mixture of above and below
3.5–4.0	Moderately participative	Group decides on basis of boss's suggestions, rules are few, group proceeds as they see fit	Independent worker, doesn't need close supervision, just a bit of feedback
4.1 and up	Very democratic	Group is in charge of decisions; boss is coordinator, group makes any rules	Self-starter, likes to challenge new things by him/herself

It should be noted that scores on this instrument will vary depending on mood and circumstances. Your leadership or followership style is best described by the range of scores from several different test times.

APPENDIX D

Test Plan for the NCLEX-PN and Test-Taking Skills

The test plan of the National Council of State Boards of Nursing, Inc. for the NCLEX-PN (National Council Licensure Examination for Practical Nurses) encompasses eight categories of practical/vocational nursing activities. Each category is vital to the assurance of the final intent of the examination: to protect the public through safe practitioners. The eight categories as given in the actual test plan, including the percent of questions allocated to each category on the examination, are listed on the following page.

◆   **Test Plan for the National Council Licensure Examination for Practical Nurses**

As of April 1994 the NCLEX-PN will be administered through computerized adaptive testing (CAT). The two major components of the test plan are the phases of the nursing process and client needs.

Nursing process

  I. Data collection (30%)
The collection of data in clients with predictable outcomes, which contributes to a data base and assists in the formulation of a nursing diagnosis.
 II. Planning (20%)
Contributes to the nursing care plan by assisting in setting goals, identifying client needs (some of which may require a change in the plan of care), and communicating with all those involved in the patient's care.
III. Implementation (30%)
Performs basic therapeutic and preventative nursing measures in a safe and effective environment. The measures follow a prescribed plan to achieve established goals, including appropriate data reporting and documenting, and assistance to the client, family, and other members of the health team in understanding the plan of care.
IV. Evaluation (20%)
Participates in evaluating effectiveness of care, observing and documenting client response to care, and how/if identified outcomes have been realized.

Client needs

  I. Safe, effective environment (24%-30%)
Includes coordinated care, standards of care, goal-oriented care, environmental safety, preparation for treatments and procedures, and safe and effective treatments and procedures.
 II. Physiologic integrity (42%-48%)
Includes physiologic adaptation, reduction of risk potential, mobility, and comfort provisions of basic care.
III. Psychosocial integrity (7%-13%)
Includes psychosocial adaptation and coping skills.
IV. Health promotion/maintenance (15%-21%)
Includes continued growth and development, self-care, integrity of support system, and prevention and early treatment of disease.

From NCLEX-PN Test Plan for National Council Licensure Examination for Practical Nurses, 1989. From Yannes-Eyles M: *Mosby's comprehensive review of practical nursing*, ed 11, St Louis, 1994, Mosby.

◆ Test-Taking Skills

Begin with a positive attitude about yourself, your nursing knowledge, and your test-taking abilities. A positive attitude is achieved through self-confidence gained by studying effectively. One of the keys to taking this exam is to "overstudy" throughout the year. Do not try to cram for the test.

Be emotionally prepared for the examination. Get a good night's sleep. In the morning allow yourself plenty of time to dress, have breakfast, and arrive at the testing site a few minutes early. Practicing a few relaxation techniques may also prove helpful to you.

Listen to the examiner and read the written directions carefully. Failure to listen or read the directions thoroughly may result in an incorrect answer, which could cause you considerable loss of points. If you have any question regarding the directions, ask the examiner for clarification.

Answer *all* questions. You are scored on the number of questions you answer correctly, not on how many you answer wrong. You have at least a 25% chance of selecting the correct answer.

Remember the time factor involved, so do not spend an excessive amount of time on any one question. One minute should be the maximum time allotted to any question. If you find it necessary to move on, make a note of the question and return to it later.

Each question contains a stem (the main intent of the question), followed by four plausible answers or alternatives that either complete a statement or answer the question presented. Only one of the alternatives is the *best* answer; the remaining alternatives are known as distractors because they are written in such a way that they could be the correct answer and distract you to a certain degree. Therefore answer each question carefully.

Read, do not scan, the situation and question carefully, looking for key words or phrases.

Key words or phrases in the stem of the question, such as first, primary, early, and best, are important. Likewise, words such as only, always, never, and all in the alternatives are frequently evidence of a wrong response.

Have confidence in your initial response to a question; it is probably the correct answer. If you are unable to answer immediately, eliminate the alternatives you know are incorrect and proceed from there. This increases your chances of randomly selecting the correct answer.

Many times the correct answer is the longest alternative given; however, do not count on it. Individuals who prepare the examination are also aware of this fact and avoid offering you any "helpful hints."

Avoid looking for an answer pattern or code. Many times, four or five consecutive questions have the same letter or number for the correct answer.

Be alert for grammatical inconsistencies. If the response is intended to complete the stem (an incomplete sentence) but makes no grammatical sense to you, it can be considered to be a distractor rather than the correct answer. However, great effort is expended by test developers to eliminate such inconsistencies.

Adapted from Yannes-Eyles M: *Mosby's comprehensive review of practical nursing,* ed 11, St Louis, 1994, Mosby.

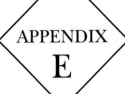

APPENDIX E

U.S., Territorial, and Canadian Nurse Licensing Bodies

◆ U.S. and Territorial Boards of Nursing

Shirley J. Dykes Silverman, Executive Officer
Board of Nursing
770 Washington Ave.
Montgomery, Alabama 36130
(205) 242-4060

Gail McGuill, RN, Executive Secretary
Alaska Board of Nursing
3601 C St., Suite 722
Anchorage, Alaska 99503
(907) 561-2878

E. B. U. Malea, RN, Secretary
Health Services Regulatory Board
LBJ Tropical Medical Center
Pago Pago, American Samoa 96799
(684) 633-1222

Fran Roberts, Executive Director
Arizona State Board of Nursing
2001 W. Camelback, Suite 350
Phoenix, Arizona 85015
(602) 255-5092

Linda Murphey, Executive Director
Arkansas State Board of Nursing
1123 South University, Suite 800
Little Rock, Arkansas 72204
(501) 371-2700

Billie Haynes, Executive Officer
Board of Vocational Nurse and Psych. Tech. Examiners
1414 K St., Suite 103
Sacramento, California 95814
(916) 324-2528

Karen Brumley, Administrator
Colorado State Board of Nursing
1560 Broadway, Suite 670
Denver, Colorado 80202
(303) 894-2435

Marie Hilliard, PhD, Executive Officer
Department of Health Services
150 Washington St.
Hartford, Connecticut 06106
(203) 566-1041

Iva J. Boardman, Executive Director
Delaware Board of Nursing
O'Neill Bldg., P.O. Box 1401
Dover, Delaware 19901
(302) 739-4522

Barbara Hatcher, Chair
District of Columbia Board of Nursing
614 H St., N.W.
Washington, DC 20013
(202) 727-7468

Judie K. Ritter, Executive Director
Florida State Board of Nursing
111 E. Coastline Dr. East
Jacksonville, Florida 32202
(904) 359-6339

Patricia N. Swann, Executive Director
Georgia Board of Examiners of Licensed
   Practical Nurses
166 Pryor St., S.W.
Atlanta, Georgia 30303
(404) 656-3921

Tina Blas, Acting Administrator
Guam Board of Nurse Examiners
P.O. Box 2816
Agana, Guam 96910
(671) 734-7296

Kathy Yokouchi, Executive Secretary
Hawaii Board of Nursing
Box 3469
Honolulu, Hawaii 99503
(808) 548-7471

Sandra E. Davis, Assistant Executive Director
Idaho State Board of Nursing
280 N. 8th St., #210
Boise, Idaho 83720
(208) 334-3110

Judy Jondahl, Nursing Education Coordinator
Department of Professional Regulation
320 W. Washington St.
Springfield, Illinois 62786
(217) 785-9465

Barbara Powers, Board Administrator
Indiana State Board of Nursing
1 American Square, Box 82067
Room 1020
Indianapolis, Indiana 46282
(317) 232-2960

Lorinda Inman, Executive Director
Iowa Board of Nursing
1223 E. Court Ave.
Des Moines, Iowa 50319
(515) 281-4828

**Lois Rich Scibetta, PhD, Executive
   Administrator**
Kansas State Board of Nursing
900 S.W. Jackson St., Suite 551S
Topeka, Kansas 66612-1256
(913) 296-3782

Sharon M. Weisenbeck, Executive Director
Kentucky Board of Nursing
4010 Dupont Circle, Suite 430
Louisville, Kentucky 40207
(502) 897-5143

Terry L. Demarcay, Executive Director
Louisiana State Board of Practical Nurse
   Examiners
1440 Canal St., Suite 1722
New Orleans, Louisiana 70112
(504) 568-6480

Jean C. Caron, Executive Director
Maine State Board of Nursing
35 Anthony Ave. St. House Sta. 158
Augusta, Maine 04333-0158
(207) 624-5275

Donna Dorsey, Executive Director
Maryland Board of Nursing
4201 Patterson Ave.
Baltimore, Maryland 21215
(301) 764-4738

Theresa M. Bonanno, Executive Secretary
Board of Registration in Nursing
100 Cambridge St., Room 150
Boston, Massachusetts 02202
(617) 727-9961

Marty Martin, Nursing Consultant
Michigan Board of Nursing
P.O. Box 30018, 611 West Ottawa
Lansing, Michigan 48909
(517) 373-1600

Joyce M. Schowalter, Executive Director
Minnesota Board of Nursing
2700 University Ave. West 108
St. Paul, Minnesota 55114
(612) 642-0575

Doris Jackson, Supervisor
Health Occupations Education Division of
   Vocational Education
Department of Education, P.O. Box 771
Jackson, Mississippi 39205
(601) 359-3938

Florence Stillman, RN, Executive Director
Missouri State Board of Nursing
3523 N. Ten Mile Dr., P.O. Box 656
Jefferson City, Missouri 65102
(314) 751-0080

Dianne Wickham, Executive Director
Montana State Board of Nursing
111 Jackson, Arcade Bldg.
Helena, Montana 59620-0407
(406) 444-4279

Charlene Kelley, PhD, Associate Director
Bureau of Examining Board
P.O. Box 95007
Lincoln, Nebraska 68509
(402) 471-2115

Mickey Wade, Associate Executive Director
Nevada State Board of Nursing
1281 Terminal Way, Room 116
Reno, Nevada 89502
(702) 786-2778

Doris G. Nuttelman, EdD, Executive Director
State Board of Nursing
Division of Public Health, 6 Hazen Dr.
Concord, New Hampshire 03301
(603) 271-2323

Sr. Teresa L. Harris, Executive Director
New Jersey Board of Nursing
P.O. Box 45010
Newark, New Jersey 07101
(201) 504-6430

Nancy L. Twigg, Executive Director
New Mexico Board of Nursing
4253 Montgomery, N.E., Suite 130
Albuquerque, New Mexico 87109
(505) 841-8340

Melene A. Megel, PhD, Executive Secretary
New York State Board for Nursing
The Cultural Center, Room 3013
Albany, New York 12230
(518) 486-2967

Carol A. Osman, Executive Director
Board of Nursing
P.O. Box 2129
Raleigh, North Carolina 27602
(919) 782-3211

Karen Macdonald, Executive Director
North Dakota Board of Nursing
919 S. 7th St., Suite 504
Bismarck, North Dakota 58504-5881
(701) 224-2974

Rosa Lee Weinert, Executive Director
Ohio Board of Nursing
77 S. High St., 17th Floor
Columbus, Ohio 43266-0316
(614) 466-3947

Sulinda Moffett, Executive Director
Oklahoma Board of Nursing
2915 N. Classen Blvd., Suite 524
Oklahoma City, Oklahoma 73106
(405) 525-2076

Joan C. Bouchard, Executive Director
Oregon State Board of Nursing
800 N.E. Oregon St. #25
Portland, Oregon 97232
(503) 644-2767

Miriam H. Limo, Executive Secretary
Pennsylvania State Board of Nurse Examiners
P.O. Box 2649
Harrisburg, Pennsylvania 17105
(717) 783-7142

Maria Alonso, Director
Department of Education Practical Nursing
    Accreditation
Box 759
Hato Rey, Puerto Rico 00919
(809) 754-9605

Patricia Molloy, Director
Board of Registration in Nursing
3 Capital Hill
Providence, Rhode Island 02908-5097
(401) 277-2827

Renatta Loquist, Executive Director
State Board of Nursing for South Carolina
220 Executive Center Dr., Suite 220
Columbia, South Carolina 29210
(803) 731-1648

Diana Vander Woude, Executive Secretary
South Dakota Board of Nursing
3307 S. Lincoln
Sioux Falls, South Dakota 57105
(605) 335-4973

Elizabeth J. Lund, RN, Executive Director
Tennessee Board of Nursing
283 Plus Park Blvd.
Nashville, Tennessee 37217
(615) 367-6264

Marjorie A. Bronk, Executive Director
Board of Vocational Nurse Examiners
9101 Burnet Rd., Suite 105
Austin, Texas 79758
(512) 835-2071

Valaine Pack, Executive Secretary
Utah State Board of Nursing
160 E. 300 South, Box 45802
Salt Lake City, Utah 84145
(801) 530-6628

Claire de Francois, Executive Director
Vermont Board of Nursing, Licensing and
    Registration Division
109 State St.
Montpelier, Vermont 05602
(802) 828-3180

Winifred Garfield, Executive Secretary
Virgin Islands Board of Nurse Licensure
P.O. Box 7309
St. Thomas, Virgin Islands 00801
(809) 776-7397

Corinne F. Dorsey, Executive Director
Virginia State Board of Nursing
1601 Rolling Hills Dr.
Richmond, Virginia 23229
(804) 662-9909

Susan L. Boots, Executive Secretary
State Board of Practical Nursing
1300 Quince St., Ey-27
Olympia, Washington 98504
(206) 753-2807

Nancy K. Wilson, Executive Secretary
Board of Examiners for Practical Nurses
922 Quarrier St., Suite 506
Charleston, West Virginia 25301
(304) 348-3572

Ramona Weakland Warden, Director
Wisconsin State Bureau of Health Service
    Professions
P.O. Box 8935
Madison, Wisconsin 53708-8935
(608) 267-2357

Toma Nisbet, Executive Director
State of Wyoming Board of Nursing
2301 Central Ave., Barrett Bldg.
Cheyenne, Wyoming 82002
(307) 777-7601

◆ Canadian Practical Nurse and Nursing Assistant Licensing Bodies

Registrar
Professional Council of Registered Nursing
    Assistants
10614-170th Street
Edmonton, Alberta
T5S 1P3

Registrar
British Columbia Council of Practical Nurses
3405 Willingdon Avenue, Room B-118
Burnaby, British Columbia
V5G 3H4
(604) 660-5750

Registrar
Manitoba Association of Licensed Practical
  Nurses
615 Kernaghan Avenue
Winnipeg, Manitoba
R2C 2Z4
(204) 222-6743

Registrar
Association of New Brunswick Registered
  Nursing Assistants
384 Smythe Street
Fredericton, New Brunswick
E3B 3E4
(506) 454-0747

Registrar
Council for Nursing Assistants
278 Kenmount Road
St. John's, Newfoundland
A1B 3R2

Registrar
Administrative Services Division
Department of Education
Government of Northwest Territories
Northway Building, 2nd Floor
Yellowknife, Northwest Territories
X1A 2L9

**Nova Scotia Board of Registration of Nursing
  Assistants**
404-2021 Brunswick Street
Halifax, Nova Scotia
B3K 2X5
(902) 423-8517

College of Nurses of Ontario
101 Davenport Road
Toronto, Ontario
M5R 3P1
(416) 928-0900
1-800-387-5526

**P.E.I. (Prince Edward Island) Licensed
  Nursing Assistants Association**
P.O. Box 1254
Charlottetown, P.E.I.
C1A 7M8
(902) 566-1512

Présidente
La Corporation professionnelle des infirmières
  et infirmiers auxiliaires du Québec
531 est, rue Sherbrooke
Montréal, Québec
H2L 1K2
(514) 282-9511

Registrar
Saskatchewan Nursing Assistants Association
2310 Smith Street
Regina, Saskatchewan
S4P 2P6
(306) 525-1436

Vicki Hancock
Registrar
Yukon Government of Justice
J-6, P.O. Box 2703
Whitehorse, Yukon
Y1A 2C6

Approved Nursing Diagnoses (North American Nursing Diagnosis Association, 1992)

Activity intolerance

Activity intolerance, high risk for

Adjustment, impaired

Airway clearance, ineffective

Anxiety

Aspiration, high risk for

Body image disturbance

Body temperature, altered, high risk for

Breastfeeding, effective

Breastfeeding, ineffective

Breastfeeding, interrupted

Breathing pattern, ineffective

Cardiac output, decreased

Caregiver role strain

Caregiver role strain, high risk for

Communication, impaired verbal

Constipation

Constipation, colonic

Constipation, perceived

Coping, defensive

Coping, family: potential for growth

Coping, ineffective family: compromised

Coping, ineffective family: disabling

Coping, ineffective individual

Decisional conflict (specify)

Denial, ineffective

Diarrhea

Disuse syndrome, high risk for

Diversional activity deficit

Dysreflexia

Family processes, altered

Fatigue

Fear

Fluid volume deficit (1)

Fluid volume deficit (2)

Fluid volume deficit, high risk for

Fluid volume excess

Gas exchange, impaired

Grieving, anticipatory

Grieving, dysfunctional

Growth and development, altered

Health maintenance, altered

Health seeking behavior (specify)

Home maintenance management, impaired

Hopelessness

Hyperthermia

Hypothermia

Incontinence, bowel

Incontinence, functional

Incontinence, reflex

Incontinence, stress

Incontinence, total

Incontinence, urge

Infant feeding pattern, ineffective

Infection, high risk for

Injury, high risk for

Knowledge deficit (specify)

Mobility, impaired physical

Noncompliance (specify)

Nutrition, altered: less than body requirements

Nutrition, altered: high risk for more than body requirements

Nutrition, altered: more than body requirements

Oral mucous membrane, altered

Pain

Pain, chronic

Parental role conflict

Parenting, altered

Parenting, altered, high risk for

Peripheral neurovascular dysfunction, high risk for

Personal identity disturbance

Poisoning, high risk for

Post-trauma response

Powerlessness

Protection, altered

Rape-trauma syndrome

Rape-trauma syndrome: compound reaction

Rape-trauma syndrome: silent reaction

Role performance, altered

Self-care deficit, bathing/hygiene

Self-care deficit, dressing/grooming

Self-care deficit, feeding

Self-care deficit, toileting

Self-esteem, chronic low

Self-esteem, disturbance

Self-esteem, situational low

Self-mutilation, high risk for

Sensory, perceptual alterations (specify: visual, auditory, kinesthetic, gustatory, tactile, olfactory)

Sexual dysfunction

Sexuality patterns, altered

Skin integrity, impaired

Skin integrity, impaired, high risk for

Sleep pattern disturbance

Social interaction, impaired

Social isolation

Spiritual distress (distress of the human spirit)

Stress syndrome, relocation

Suffocation, high risk for

Swallowing, impaired

Therapeutic regimen (individual), ineffective management of

Thermoregulation, ineffective

Thought processes, altered

Tissue integrity, impaired

Tissue perfusion, altered (specify: renal, cerebral, cardiopulmonary, gastrointestinal, peripheral)

Trauma, high risk for

Unilateral neglect

Urinary elimination, altered patterns

Urinary retention

Ventilation, spontaneous inability to sustain

Ventilatory weaning response, dysfunctional (DVWR)

Violence, high risk for self-directed or directed at others

Index

Page numbers in italics indicate illustrations; *t* indicates tables.